Gil G. Noam
Editor-in-Chief

NEW DIRECTIONS FOR YOUTH DEVELOPMENT

Theory
Practice
Research

fall | 2006

Preparing Youth for the Crossing

From Adolescence to Early Adulthood

Sam Piha
Georgia Hall

issue editors

JOSSEY-BASS ™
An Imprint of
WILEY

PREPARING YOUTH FOR THE CROSSING: FROM ADOLESCENCE TO EARLY ADULTHOOD
Sam Piha, Georgia Hall (eds.)
New Directions for Youth Development, No. 111, Fall 2006
Gil G. Noam, Editor-in-Chief

Microfilm copies of issues and articles are available in 16mm and 35mm, as well as microfiche in 105mm, through University Microfilms Inc., 300 North Zeeb Road, Ann Arbor, Michigan 48106-1346.

NEW DIRECTIONS FOR YOUTH DEVELOPMENT (ISSN 1533-8916, electronic ISSN 1537-5781) is part of The Jossey-Bass Psychology Series and is published quarterly by Wiley Subscription Services, Inc., A Wiley Company, at Jossey-Bass, 989 Market Street, San Francisco, California 94103-1741. POSTMASTER: Send address changes to New Directions for Youth Development, Jossey-Bass, 989 Market Street, San Francisco, California 94103-1741.

SUBSCRIPTIONS cost $80.00 for individuals and $195.00 for institutions, agencies, and libraries. Prices subject to change. Refer to the order form at the back of this issue.

EDITORIAL CORRESPONDENCE should be sent to the Editor-in-Chief, Dr. Gil G. Noam, McLean Hospital, 115 Mill Street, Belmont, MA 02478.

Cover photograph by Veer

www.josseybass.com

Contents

Editors' Notes

THE TRANSITION OF YOUTH from adolescence to early adulthood has historically been marked by graduation from high school, followed by decisions to pursue higher education or vocational training, or move directly into the labor market or military—all with the goal of becoming economically self-sufficient. Today, however, there is growing concern that for large numbers of older youth, particularly low-income youth of color, these milestones are becoming increasingly difficult to achieve. Furthermore, as a society, we are not offering young people ages fourteen and older the supports and opportunities they need to acquire the knowledge, skills, and practical experiences to make this transition successfully. Public high schools often fail to engage their students, and a high percentage of youth, especially black and Hispanic youth, drop out of school early or fail to earn their high school diplomas. At the same time, members of the business community report that an alarming number of students who do graduate lack the basic skills required in the workplace.

Over the past forty years, there have been significant investments, both public and private, in programs that seek to improve outcomes for children. The 1965 launch and subsequent growth of the Head Start program and the more recent expansion of the 21st Century Community Learning Centers were significant victories for the advocates of low-income children and families. However, most of these new investments focused on the needs of young children. There are few policy initiatives that focus on or acknowledge the needs of older youth or offer the resources to better prepare

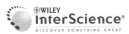

young people for the challenges of early adulthood before they age out of the educational system.

In order to see improved outcomes for older youth, particularly low-income youth of color, we need to focus our attention on their needs now. For these young people, the clock is ticking; they deserve a better chance to succeed. To better serve their needs, we need a shared knowledge and understanding of what their developmental needs are and the challenges they face in meeting these needs in today's world.

We need to improve both in-school and out-of-school experiences to make learning more engaging and relevant to youths' lives. We need to also promote both expansion of and innovation in out-of-school-time programs so we can attract and engage more youth in developing their interests and skills that will be relevant to them after high school. This cannot happen without policies that call for increased funding and technical assistance to high schools and community programs that serve older youth, better coordination and collaboration at the systems levels, and the reform of policies that impede rather than support efforts to better prepare youth for transition to adulthood.

We hope this issue of *New Directions for Youth Development* will bring increased focus on the needs of older youth and offer ideas and working models for how we can better prepare them for the road ahead.

In Chapter One, Nicole Zarrett and Jacquelynne Eccles explain the major developmental changes and challenges associated with late adolescence. They point to the critical importance of understanding the supports older youth need to stay on healthy, positive trajectories. By blending developmental theory and youth development research findings, the authors provide valuable insight into the transition from adolescence to adulthood.

In Chapter Two, Marion Goldstein and Pedro Noguera review the challenges and hardships faced by low-income urban youth of color that place them at risk and shape their lives and the opportunities available to them. While prevention programs present one strategy to help urban youth avoid the risk of substance abuse, most are ineffective because they are not tailored to meet the cultural sensibilities of diverse adolescent populations. Goldstein and

Noguera present an alternative strategy relevant to any program serving this population—one that places diversity with respect to culture, class, and environment at the center of program efforts.

In Chapter Three, Georgia Hall discusses the urgency of integrating technology skill building into youth development experiences. The chapter outlines race, gender, and socioeconomic differences among teens in technology access and utilization and ends with recommended approaches for ensuring that all teens have access to the knowledge and skills needed to meet the demands of the twenty-first century.

The next two chapters focus on school-based initiatives and the potential of school reform and high school after-school programs to promote youth engagement and support school success. In Chapter Four, James Connell and Adena Klem describe the Institute for Research and Reform in Education's development of First Things First (FTF), a school reform framework grounded in youth development research. Independent evaluation has confirmed that the use of the framework in schools serving large numbers of minority and economically disadvantaged students is associated with higher persistence and graduation rates and better performance on state tests. The authors stress the need for adults in schools to build better relationships with students and employ strategies to increase the personalization of their education. They detail four critical features within the FTF framework that are focused on students and discuss three specific strategies for achieving these features in schools.

In Chapter Five, Sarah Barr, Jennifer Birmingham, Jennifer Fornal, Rachel Klein, and Sam Piha review the insights and lessons learned from three after-school initiatives: the After School Safety and Education for Teens, After School Matters, and the After-School Corporation. Although each of these programs has a different structure, all have shown success in attracting high school students to their programs and engaging them in meaningful activities to support their success in school and transition to early adulthood. The chapter ends with recommendations for policymakers and funders related to funding, accountability, program quality, and diverse learning opportunities.

Chapter Six, by Joan Arches and Jennie Fleming, presents two case studies of youth projects in the United Kingdom and United

States that demonstrate the use of social action as a viable program approach to encourage youth participation and civic engagement. The Young People's Research and Development Project (United Kingdom) and the Healthy Initiative Collaborative (United States) provide opportunities for youth to become community researchers and problem solvers and thus contribute to community change in ways that are meaningful and empowering to them. Comments from youth in the chapter add to our understanding of the value of a social action approach and the variety of outcomes, including self-awareness, self-reflection, and skill mastery, it can stimulate.

In Chapter Seven, David Brown and Mala Thakur report on the challenges facing youth who are disconnected from our nation's employment and education systems. They share insights into the various strategies that have been implemented to facilitate the transition of older youth to the workforce and feature the work of the Promising and Effective Practices Network to develop tools designed to help organizations develop quality programs that connect youth to jobs, careers, and education.

In Chapter Eight, Mark Ouellette highlights the importance of developing a communitywide approach to supporting the needs of older youth. The need for out-of-school-time supports and opportunities does not disappear with age. Ouellette suggests that the following system-level components are essential to a successful program: an understanding of what youth want, communitywide leadership with an effective plan, coordination among key stakeholders, high school programming standards that include youth voice, and coordinated and adequate funding.

In the final chapter, Nicole Yohalem, Alicia Wilson-Ahlstrom, Thaddeus Ferber, and Elizabeth Gaines focus on five issues that demonstrate how policies related to out-of-school time can be aligned with the developmental needs of older youth: financial incentives, school credit, alternative pathways to credentials, participation requirements, and funding. This final chapter reminds us that preparing young people for the future requires the full engagement of all community institutions, small and large, public and private, in supporting learning and development.

NEW DIRECTIONS FOR YOUTH DEVELOPMENT • DOI: 10.1002/yd

This volume delineates the complexities and urgency of supporting older youth as they make the transition from late adolescence to adulthood—their challenges, the skills they need, and the surrounding environment. The good news, as noted in this volume, is that there are many innovative and effective initiatives forging a path forward on which we can continue to build.

Sam Piha
Georgia Hall
Editors

SAM PIHA *is the director for community and school partnerships at Community Network for Youth Development in San Francisco.*

GEORGIA HALL *is a research scientist at the National Institute on Out-of-School Time, part of the Wellesley Centers for Women at Wellesley College.*

Executive Summary

Chapter One: The passage to adulthood: Challenges of late adolescence

Nicole Zarrett, Jacquelynne Eccles

Late adolescence and the period following, often referred to as emerging adulthood, have been noted as particularly important for setting the stage for continued development through the life span as individuals begin to make choices and engage in a variety of activities that are influential for the rest of their lives. Demographic, sociocultural, and labor market changes have made the years between ages eighteen and twenty-five more transitional than in the recent past. This chapter reviews the critical assets and needs that are essential for keeping youth on healthy, productive pathways into adulthood and examines the developmental tasks and changes of late adolescence.

Chapter Two: Designing for diversity: Incorporating cultural competence in prevention programs for urban youth

Marion J. Goldstein, Pedro A. Noguera

Low-income urban youth of color frequently confront a wide variety of challenges and hardships that other young people never

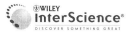

NEW DIRECTIONS FOR YOUTH DEVELOPMENT, NO. 111, FALL 2006 © WILEY PERIODICALS, INC.
Published online in Wiley InterScience (www.interscience.wiley.com) • DOI: 10.1002/yd.178

experience. The offering of prevention programs represents one strategy to help urban youth avoid the risks associated with substance abuse. In this chapter, an alternative program strategy is posited—one that places diversity with respect to culture, class, and environment at the center of prevention efforts. Such an approach, the authors argue, is more effective not only in appealing to the sensibilities of urban youth but also in altering their behavior.

Chapter Three: Teens and technology: Preparing for the future

Georgia Hall

In the past two decades, economic, technological, demographic, and political forces have stimulated major change in the learning and working landscape for young people. These circumstances compel us to prioritize the integration of technology skill building into youth development experiences in order to better prepare older youth for the challenges and responsibilities ahead. Facilitating older youth's acquisition of technology skills must continue to be a principal goal of policymakers, city leaders, and youth program providers. This chapter looks at the integration of technology skill building into youth development experiences with consideration of gender and races differences in technology access and utilization, along with challenges that at-risk teens face.

Chapter Four: First Things First: A framework for successful secondary school reform

James P. Connell, Adena M. Klem

If youth development initiatives are going to focus on outcomes that we know are important in settings that we know can change these outcomes, the first outcomes should be educational, and the first setting should be school. School reform presents the most feasible, defensible, and informed opportunity for public policy to improve the life chances of children and youth in disadvantaged communities. This chapter introduces First Things First (FTF), a school reform framework grounded in research about how young people develop and how schools promote students' engagement and learning. The chapter explores four critical features of FTF that focus on students: (1) continuity of care; (2) increased instructional time; (3) high, clear, and fair standards; and (4) enriched opportunities for students. The critical features of FTF are implemented through three strategies: small learning communities, a family advocate system, and instructional improvement.

Chapter Five: Three high school after-school initiatives: Lessons learned

Sarah Barr, Jennifer Birmingham, Jennifer Fornal, Rachel Klein, Sam Piha

Alarmed by the large numbers of high school–age youth who are disengaged at school and leaving high school without a diploma or the important skills for the workplace, policymakers and youth advocates are beginning to see high school afterschool as the new frontier in after-school programming. Although older youth represent a sizable percentage of American students, they garner only a small fraction of the federal, state, and local investments for after-school programs. This chapter reviews the insights and lessons learned from three after-school initiatives that have shown success in attracting high school students to their programs and engaging them in meaningful activities to support their success in school and transition to early adulthood: the After School Safety and Education for Teens, After School Matters, and the After-School Corporation. Emerging from these pioneering efforts are some promising practices and program models that can guide the development of future after-school programs, but not without the help of policymakers and funders, both public and private.

Chapter Six: Young people and social action: Youth participation in the United Kingdom and United States

Joan Arches, Jennie Fleming

This chapter provides two case studies of projects in the United Kingdom and United States using a social action approach to encourage youth participation and civic engagement. The authors provide a snapshot of U.K. and U.S. policy related to inclusionary practice in youth development work, along with testimony from youth participating in the two community development initiatives. As part of the positive youth development approach, youth inclusion is seen as a key to policy, programs, planning, and practice with young people. Educators, researchers, and practitioners using participatory methodologies have continued to move the youth development field forward. Social action provides a theory and practice that enhances community building, social cohesion, and positive youth development.

Chapter Seven: Workforce development for older youth

David E. Brown, Mala B. Thakur

The challenges facing youth who are disconnected from our nation's employment and education systems are expansive. Research has suggested that youth services and supports that are grounded in a developmental approach not only help young people avoid self-destructive behavior, but also enable them to acquire the academic and work-readiness skills and personal attributes that employers seek. In 1995, the National Youth Employment Coalition and its members established the Promising and Effective Practices Network (PEPNet) to identify the key elements of quality youth programs and develop tools that would help organizations establish, connect to, and promote quality programs. PEPNet represents a standards framework that captures the key elements common to successful programs that connect youth to jobs, careers, and education. This chapter provides some insights into the current practices that have been implemented to facilitate older youth's transition to the workforce and highlights the supports youth need for successful adulthood, citizenship, and career pursuits.

Chapter Eight: Going the distance: Serving the needs of older youth at scale

Mark Ouellette

Few communities have developed successful strategies for attracting large numbers of older youth to their out-of-school-time programs. In addition to meeting the unique developmental and programmatic needs of this population, communities have struggled with the challenge of creating communitywide integrated approaches to service delivery and resource development. Communities wanting to build a system of supports for older youth must do so in the context of a communitywide strategy as opposed to fragmented, individually operating programs and services. A communitywide strategy creates greater opportunity for strategic mobilization of resources, greater funding leverage, evaluation and assessment consistency, and more powerful input into creating a public voice and public will for supporting and serving older youth as they make the transition to adulthood.

Chapter Nine: Supporting older youth: What's policy got to do with it?

Nicole Yohalem, Alicia Wilson-Ahlstrom, Thaddeus Ferber, Elizabeth Gaines

The nonschool hours are an underused tool in supporting older youth in their transition to adulthood. Given competing demands on many teens' time and a host of other developmental realities, effective strategies for engaging high schoolers look much different from those of their younger counterparts, and those differences have programmatic and policy implications. Effective youth policies reflect an overarching vision that is about changing lives—a vision that addresses a range of risk and protective factors, simultaneously supports discrete programs and builds coherent pathways to success, and recognizes that children and youth grow up in families and communities. This chapter highlights policy innovations related to teens' involvement in out-of-school-time activities and then looks at three principles that can help ensure that youth policy supports the full range of older youth's unique developmental, social, and economic needs.

This chapter outlines the major developmental challenges likely to affect overall well-being during adolescence and emerging adulthood and discusses the personal and social assets needed to facilitate a successful passage through adolescence and into adulthood.

1

The passage to adulthood: Challenges of late adolescence

Nicole Zarrett, Jacquelynne Eccles

THERE ARE MAJOR developmental changes and challenges associated with the period of adolescence, as youth acquire and consolidate the competencies, attitudes, values, and social capital necessary to make a successful transition into adulthood. Late adolescence and the period following, often referred to as emerging adulthood, have been noted as particularly important for setting the stage for continued development through the life span as individuals begin to make choices and engage in a variety of activities that are influential on the rest of their lives. As youth move into emerging adulthood around the age of eighteen (often on completion of high school), their choices and challenges shift to include decisions about education or vocational training, entry into and transitions within the labor market, moving out of the family home, and sometimes marriage and parenthood. Although early adolescence has received much attention by researchers as a period of major distress, recently late adolescence has become a period of concern among developmental researchers and youth advocates.

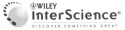

NEW DIRECTIONS FOR YOUTH DEVELOPMENT, NO. 111, FALL 2006 © WILEY PERIODICALS, INC.
Published online in Wiley InterScience (www.interscience.wiley.com) • DOI: 10.1002/yd.179

Demographic, sociocultural, and labor market changes have made the years between ages eighteen and twenty-five more transitional than in the recent past. Thirty years ago, the period of adolescence was considered to end somewhere between ages eighteen and twenty-two, at which point youth would choose between a small, easily understood set of options following high school: youth chose to move into college, the labor market, or the military and got married and had children during their early twenties. These well-defined pathways from adolescence into adulthood no longer exist for most social class groups.[1] This increased complexity and heterogeneity in the passage into adulthood make the late adolescent period more challenging than in the past, especially for non-college-bound youth and members of several ethnic minority groups.

It is essential to examine the influence of structural constraints on adolescents' choices and engagement in activities that promote future options and opportunities and trajectories. It is also critical to understand what assets and needs are essential for keeping youth on healthy, productive pathways into adulthood. As Erik Erikson asserted, tasks of adolescence are played out in a complex set of social contexts and in both cultural and historical settings.[2]

Challenges

The developmental tasks of adolescence that Erikson outlined include the development of a sense of mastery, identity, and intimacy. Others have added the establishment of autonomy, management of sexuality and intimacy, and finding a niche for oneself in education and work.[3] Eccles and Gootman elaborated on these tasks, identifying several more specific challenges: (1) shifts in relationship with parents from dependency and subordination to one that reflects the adolescent's increasing maturity and responsibilities in the family and the community, (2) the exploration of new roles (both social and sexual), (3) the experience of intimate partnerships, (4) identity formation at both the social and personal levels, (5) planning one's future and taking the necessary steps to pursue those plans, and (6) acquiring the range of skills and values needed to make a successful transition into adulthood (including work, partnership, parenting, and citizenship).

By emerging adulthood, youth are increasingly independent, acquire and manage greater responsibility, and take on an active role in their own development. Eccles and Gootman go on to specify some primary challenges in this last stage of adolescence when youth begin to take on more demanding roles: (1) the management of these demanding roles, (2) identifying personal strengths and weaknesses and refining skills to coordinate and succeed in these roles, (3) finding meaning and purpose in the roles acquired, and (4) assessing and making necessary life changes and coping with these changes. Successful management of all these challenges depends on the psychosocial, physical, and cognitive assets of the individual; the social supports available; and the developmental settings in which young people can explore and interact with these challenges.[4]

Physical and biological changes

During early adolescence, youth experience dramatic changes in the shape of their bodies, an increase in gonadal hormones, and changes in brain architecture. Another major biological change during this period between puberty and young adulthood is in the frontal lobes of the brain, responsible for such functions as self-control, judgment, emotional regulation, organization, and planning.[5] These changes in turn fuel major shifts in adolescents' physical and cognitive capacities and their social and achievement-related needs. During early adolescence, the primary task consists of managing these biological and cognitive shifts and the subsequent influences these have on behavior, mood, and social relationships. How youth cope with these changes will ultimately influence their well-being in later adolescence as multiple additional tasks are imposed on them.

Cognitive development

Cognitive skill development over the adolescent years enables youth to become increasingly capable of managing their own learning and problem solving while also facilitating their identity formation and maturation of moral reasoning. There are distinct increases in adolescents' capacities to think abstractly, consider multiple dimensions of problems, process information and stimuli more efficiently, and reflect on the self and life experiences.[6]

The successful development of these cognitive skills relates to youth's ability to be planful, an important skill for successful pursuit of educational and occupational goals.[7] It has also been linked with adolescents' greater investments in understanding their own and others' internal psychological states and the resulting behavioral shift in focus on their developing close and intimate friendships. As young people consider what possibilities are available to them, they are more capable of reflecting on their own abilities, interests, desires, and needs. Overall, youth are able to come to a deeper understanding of the social and cultural settings in which they live. In fact, research has found an increase in youth's commitments to civic involvement when such cognitive developments are coupled with prosocial values and opportunities to think and discuss issues of tolerance and human interaction with others. In a culture that stresses personal choice in life planning, these concerns and interests set the stage for personal and social identity formation and ultimately influence educational, occupational, recreational, and marital and family choices.[8]

Achievement

One of the key milestones for older youth is graduation from high school.

High school

For some youth, adolescence continues to be a time for continued educational growth and success and promising goals and plans for the future. For others, adolescence is marked by major declines in academic performance, interest, and self-perceptions of ability and heightened risk for academic failure and dropout. Some researchers suggest that these declines are due to an "intrapsychic upheaval" as youth struggle to manage the simultaneous occurrence of multiple life changes.[9]

NEW DIRECTIONS FOR YOUTH DEVELOPMENT • DOI: 10.1002/yd

Other research has found that academic declines in interest and self-concept are a function of the mismatch between the school environment and the adolescent. Person-environment fit theory outlines how behavior, motivation, and mental health are influenced by the fit between the characteristics that individuals bring to their environments and characteristics of the environments themselves: whether individuals will fare well and be motivated depends on whether the social environment meets their needs. When school environments do not meet adolescents' changing needs, their academic motivation, interest, and performance will decline. Difficulties in early adolescence, with the transition into middle school, seem especially harmful, setting some youth on a downward spiral of low academic motivation and achievement throughout high school.[10]

In addition, in all Western societies, one of the most universal factors behind academic success throughout the entire educational career is socioeconomic background. For the United States, there is ample empirical evidence that socioeconomic status is the single best predictor of academic achievement from elementary school onward.[11] Schnabel, Alfeld, Eccles, Köller, and Baumert found that children from lower socioeconomic strata are not only less successful in high school, but they also have a significantly smaller empirical chance to move into a four-year full-time college education even after controlling for academic achievement and other psychological factors.[12]

The school continues to be an institution that provides youth a support network for positive development through emerging adulthood. However, youth first need confidence in their abilities, good social skills, high self-esteem, and good coping skills to manage the multiple challenges and stressors associated with the high school environment in order to gain the experiences and resources needed to pursue postsecondary education.[13]

Transition to college

At completion of high school, about half of America's youth enroll in college, and the remaining half move into a variety of work and nonwork settings.[14] This difference in transitional trajectories involves very different experiences and challenges for youth on the different tracks. Universities serve as social institutions that provide youth shelter, organized activities, adult and peer support, health care, and a various forms of entertainment. College-bound youth discover new-found independence: the college environment enables them to practice self-governance, individuation from parents, and freedom to direct their own lifestyle in a safe environment that delays many adult responsibilities.[15] As a result, college-bound youth have the opportunity to extend exploration of the self, develop new ideas, take advantage of multiple opportunities, and try out various lifestyles.[16] In essence, universities are social institutions that have become increasingly tailored to provide a sort of semiautonomy to assist the transition into young adulthood.

Although a college education has become increasingly important for ensuring a bright future, the transition into and persistence in college can be challenging and stressful. According to census data in 2000, only 52 percent of those enrolled in college are reported to receive their initial degree objective within five years.[17] Although research on college retention is in its early stages, some findings pinpoint factors that are especially important for college retention. The high dropout rates during college are related to such factors as unfamiliar academic expectations, changes in sources of social support, and social norms that encourage high levels of risky behaviors, particularly alcohol use.[18]

College enrollment and retention is especially challenging for low-income youth. Between entering college and graduating, low-socioeconomic-status (SES) students are at significantly greater risk of dropping out of college in comparison to their middle- to upper-SES counterparts.[19] Background factors such as minority status, SES, gender, and high school performance can influence commitment to college through their influence on students' integration into the social and academic structures of the institution. Therefore, along with the direct costs of college, other social and cognitive factors confounded with SES are also important to consider when examining attrition once a student arrives at college.

There are also youth who seem to be caught in the middle. They come from middle-income families but are well short of affluent.

Without qualifications for receiving support from the state and only modest help from their financially overextended families, these youth are often left to manage on their own. They often must juggle work and school responsibilities, which leads to a set of additional challenges and often to delays in attaining a college degree well into their late twenties and early thirties.[20]

Therefore, high cognitive resources, prior knowledge, and financial security are not the only factors that help adolescents make a successful adjustment to college. Research has found that family support, adolescents' personal appreciation for education and learning (interest, value, aspiration), and high academic self-concept (belief in their own competence) are just as important for supporting youth's enrollment and persistence in college.[21]

School-to-work

The other half of youth who do not enroll in some form of postsecondary education are not only deprived of educational and occupational advancements, but also the developmental moratorium of exploration and experimentation experienced by youth enrolled in college full time.[22] Approximately one out of seven youth drop out of high school, often working sporadically if employed at all, and many youth who do finish high school and move straight into work do not fare much better. There are not many institutional supports in the United States to help adolescents on this pathway, leaving them to manage the school-to-work transition almost entirely by themselves. The military and some volunteer programs have served as a few social institutions that provide a setting for youth to live, work, and learn. These programs are tailored to offer youth the opportunity to develop further skill and experience and heighten a sense of competence by providing sponsored independence: semiautonomy, expectations, and demands coupled with guidance, mentoring, and support. There are also some apprenticeships and training programs designed to provide supports.[23] However, most noncollege-bound youth do not find such supports and often end up floundering in the labor force in the hope of finding secure, well-paying employment from their late teens through their twenties. The social structure is currently so ill designed to support such a school-to-work trajectory that it results in what seems a chaotic or haphazard entry into adulthood for these youth. Such important needs as housing and medical insurance cannot be afforded at typical starting wages for high school students or graduates, and these young people cannot easily establish financial independence and an independent household. Without a college education (or additional training through the military or an apprenticeship), it is extremely difficult to make such developmental transitions, especially for those who aspire to at least a middle-class job and middle-class lifestyle.[24]

Social relationships

During adolescence, youth also must deal with changes in many of their social relationships, providing opportunities to develop and exercise their personal and social identities and further explore their autonomy.

Family relationships

Parent-child relationships are highly related to youth well-being, and maintaining strong ties to one's family is important for the adolescent and emerging adulthood years.[25] Along with school and work, the family is another institution that often provides youth with important assets for positive development. Families can give youth financial, emotional, and achievement-related support; provide social capital; and act as important role models.

Although families of origin function as a central safety net for many adolescents, they also function as a serious risk for others whose family lacks such supports. During early adolescence, there are increases in parent-child conflicts as children's needs for autonomy and independence increase and they show some resistance to family rules and roles.[26] In many Western cultures, some distancing in parent-child relationships is viewed as functional, helping youth to individualize from their parents, try more things on their own, and develop their own competence. Most of these conflicts do not concern core issues such as education, politics, or spirituality, but rather focus on minor issues such as appearance, chores, and dating. For most youth, family relationships generally improve as they move into the later adolescent years, although more serious conflicts between youth and their parents during the early adolescent years can result in more serious challenges for youth throughout adolescence.

Some youth are in family situations in which parents are unavailable, unable, or, in some cases, unwilling to provide the support their children need to make a successful transition into adulthood. These youth are often placed at high risk because of such factors as parent divorce, poverty, unemployment, death, or psychological estrangement of parents and their children.[27] For example, when poverty is coupled with living in a single-parent household as well as having a minority status, youth are at high risk for dropping out of high school, drug and alcohol abuse, smoking, violence, sexual intercourse, and gang-related behavior.[28] How families and youth manage late adolescence thus varies greatly by the resources available to them.

During adolescence, youth often establish strong relationships with adults in organized activity settings as well. Teachers, coaches, program organizers, spiritual leaders, and parents of friends all can serve as additional mentors who can help buffer the impact of poor relationships with parents or negative peer influences, as well as provide further social capital for achievement-related success.

Friendships

The peer group has been found to be a powerful place for identity formation and consolidation throughout the adolescent period.[29] One of the most major changes during adolescence is youth's increasing focus on peer relationships as indicated by increases in both the time they spend with peers and their engagement in activities done with peers. In fact, peer acceptance and time spent doing activities with peers commonly take precedence over academics during early adolescence and can result in an increase in problem behaviors if the youth are subjected to excessive peer pressure to engage in such behaviors. This may ultimately compromise youth's successful transition to adulthood.[30] However as adolescents get older and more confident in their abilities, social status, and own goals and values, the impact of peer relationships on behavior declines.[31]

Romantic partnerships

During adolescence, peers also become romantic partners. Romantic relationships are speculated to play a role in identity formation during adolescence by connecting youth with their peers and providing them a sense of belonging and status in their peer groups. In addition, dating and romantic relationships during adolescence are positively related to feelings of self-worth, and longitudinal evidence indicates that by late adolescence, feeling competent in romantic relationships contributes largely to general feelings of competence.[32]

Although the development of romantic relations is another means for developing one's identity and exploring adult roles, such rising romantic and sexual interests during adolescence are also accompanied by an increase in risks of teenage pregnancy and sexually transmitted diseases. Sexual behaviors increase dramatically during adolescence. A report from the National Longitudinal Study of Adolescent Health indicates that rates of sexual intercourse rise from 16 percent among seventh and eighth graders to 60 percent among eleventh and twelfth graders.[33] The rate of age-related increases in sexual intercourse is especially high among youth who are involved in extended romantic relationships and who see the benefits of sexual relations as high and the cost of sexual relations (including pregnancy) as low. Rates are low among youth who want to avoid becoming pregnant so they can achieve their educational and occupational aspirations. In fact, research suggests that having opportunities and aspirations for attaining prestigious education and career trajectories helps youth negotiate their romantic and sexual relations and their achievement-related roles.[34]

Implications

This chapter has outlined the major developmental challenges likely to affect overall well-being during adolescence and emerging adulthood. Some youth develop a set of personal assets that help them successfully meet these challenges and develop the skills, attitudes, values, and social capital they need for a successful transition into adulthood. Developmental theorists have identified several specific personal assets believed to be most critical for healthy development. These include having confidence in one's ability to achieve one's goals and make a difference in the world and strong desires to engage in important activities (intrinsic motivation), master learning tasks, and be socially connected. Youth also need to develop the ability to control and regulate their emotions, have a sense of optimism, and develop attachment to and engagement in at least one or two conventional prosocial institutions: schools, faith-based organizations, families, and community organizations, for example.[35] Murnane and Levy stress how such assets are also important for successful entry into the labor market.[36]

Although most youth have some of these personal assets to deal with the challenges at least somewhat effectively, many have not been given the same opportunities to acquire such assets and thus flounder throughout the adolescent and emerging-adulthood years. How can we design our social institutions and policies to better match adolescents' shifts in needs? How can we improve the personal skills and resources of today's youth so that more youth successfully navigate and manage the transition to adulthood? Out-of-school activity settings is one means by which youth may find the support and resources they need to help smooth their transition into adulthood.[37]

During early and middle adolescence, not only do almost all youth attend school, but many of these same youth also receive additional support from youth organizations. By late adolescence, these supports either diverge or disappear altogether. As youth develop, family conflict common during the early adolescent years decreases, as does susceptibility to peer influence. Biological systems stabilize, cognitive skills increase, and expertise in various domains grows. Both personal and social identity concerns increase, especially those related to occupational, sexual, and ethnic identities. Therefore, programs and institutions developed to cater to the needs of older youth must map onto their growing maturity and expertise, the new courses they are taking in high school, their increasing cognitive capacities, their increased concerns about identity issues, and their movement toward adulthood.[38]

Community programs have the potential to provide a safe setting for youth to explore themselves, their interests, and their abilities in a wide range of activities and among a diversity of people. Such experiences can aid youth in dealing with issues regarding their social identity development as well as nurture tolerance and respect for diversity.

Community organizations can function to counteract the experiences in many schools that undermine adolescents' academic motivation and school engagement. These programs should therefore focus on nurturing youth's new cognitive skills and help youth form positive, realistic views of themselves in order to make well-informed decisions and plans. Especially for older adolescents, programs should stress future plans and support high educational and occupational goals. Not only will this help guide youth onto successful educational and career paths, but some interventions designed to help youth form and maintain high educational and occupation goals and reduce involvement in romantic relationships have been effective at lowering rates of unprotected sexual activity and unplanned pregnancies.[39]

Relationships are primary supports that help youth navigate adolescence and the transition to adulthood. Therefore, there is also a strong need for building and supporting family relationships and resources. As adolescents age, community programs can help facilitate positive, supportive relationships with both familial and nonfamilial adults in which youth can discuss important issues of identity and morality and future life plans and goals. Along with the importance of having young adult mentors for youth to look up to as ideal examples of successful transitions into adulthood, providing opportunities for these older adolescents to work with and supervise younger adolescents is just as important, giving older adolescents the feeling of being respected and that they are making an important contribution. Finally, as pressure from peers to engage in problem behaviors increases throughout adolescence, there is a rising need for programs to create and support positive peer groups to help youth develop strong social and personal identities.[40]

Programs need to be developmentally appropriate by providing opportunity for increasing autonomy and allowing youth to participate in program decision making and leadership, as well as by exposing youth to intellectually and cognitively challenging material. Eccles and Gootman suggest that programs for older youth should involve (1) an educational element that helps youth prepare for college courses, learn about multiple cultures, and develop the skills to navigate across multiple cultural settings; (2) opportunities to mentor younger adolescents and take on leadership roles; and (3) aid youth in focusing on their educational and career goals through providing career-related experiences in a variety of occupational settings and career planning activities. In combination, such supports will help young people develop personal strategies of success.[41]

Notes

1. Furstenberg, F., Rumbaut, R. G., & Settersten, R. A. (2005). On the frontier of adulthood: An introduction. In R. A. Settersten, F. Furstenberg, & R. G. Rumbaut (Eds.), *On the frontier of adulthood: Theory, research, and public policy* (pp. 3–28). Chicago: University of Chicago Press.

2. Erikson, E. (1968). *Identity: Youth and crisis*. New York: Norton; Bronfenbrenner, U. (1979). T*he ecology of human development: Experiments by nature and design*. Cambridge, MA: Harvard University Press; Eccles, J. S., Midgley, C., Buchanan, C. M., Wigfield, A., Reuman, D., & MacIver, D. (1993). Development during adolescence: The impact of stage/environment fit. *American Psychologist, 48*, 90–101.

3. Carnegie Corporation of New York. (1989). *Turning points: Preparing American youth for the 21st century*. New York: Author; Havinghurst, R. J. (1972). *Developmental tasks and education*. New York: McKay.

4. Eccles, J. S., & Gootman, J. A. (Eds.). (2002). *Community Programs to Promote Youth Development/Committee on Community-Level Programs for Youth*. Washington, DC: National Academy Press; Eccles, J. S., Templeton, J., Barber, B., & Stone, M. (2003). Adolescence and emerging adulthood: The critical passage ways to adulthood. In M. H. Bornstein, L. Davidson, C. Keyes, & K. A. Moore (Eds.), *Positive development across the life course* (pp. 383–406). Mahwah, NJ: Erlbaum.

5. Begley, S. (2000, Feb. 28). Getting inside a teen brain: Hormones aren't the only reason adolescents act crazy. Their gray matter differs from children's and adults'. *Newsweek*, 58–59.

6. Keating, D. P. (1990). Adolescent thinking. In S. S. Feldman & G. R. Elliot (Eds.), *At the threshold: The developing adolescent* (pp. 54–89). Cambridge, MA: Harvard University Press; Wigfield, A., Eccles, J. S., & Pintrich, P. R. (1996). Development between the ages of eleven and twenty-five. In D. C. Berliner & R. C. Calfee (Eds.), *The handbook of educational psychology* (pp. 148–185). New York: Macmillan.

7. Heckhausen, J. (1999). *Developmental regulation in adulthood.* Cambridge: Cambridge University Press.

8. Furstenberg, Rumbaut, & Settersten. (2005).

9. Simmons, R. G., & Blyth, D. A. (1987). *Moving into adolescence: The impact of pubertal change and school context.* Hawthorne, NY: Aldine de Gruyter; Arnett, J. J. (1999). Adolescent storm and stress, reconsidered. *American Psychologist, 54,* 317–326.

10. Eccles, J. S., Midgley, C., Buchanan, C. M., Wigfield, A., Reuman, D., & MacIver, D. (1993). Development during adolescence: The impact of stage/environment fit. *American Psychologist, 48,* 90–101; Eccles, J. S., Wigfield, A., & Schiefele, U. (1998). Motivation to succeed. In N. Eisenberg (Vol. Ed.), *Handbook of child psychology: Social, emotional, and personality development* (5th ed., pp. 1017–1095). Hoboken, NJ: Wiley.

11. Duncan, G., & Brooks-Gunn, J. (1997). *Consequences of growing up poor.* New York: Russell Sage Foundation.

12. Schnabel, K. U., Alfeld, C., Eccles, J. S., Köller, O., & Baumert, J. (2002). Parental influence on students' educational choices in the United States and Germany: Different ramifications—same effect? *Journal of Vocational Behavior, 60*(2), 178–198.

13. Lord, S. E., Eccles, J. S., & McCarthy, K. A. (1994). Surviving the junior high school transition: Family processes and self-perceptions as protective and risk factors. *Journal of Early Adolescence, 14,* 162–199.

14. William T. Grant Foundation. (1988). *The forgotten half: Pathways to success for America's youth and young families.* Washington, DC: William T. Grant Commission on Work, Family, and Citizenship.

15. Flanagan, C., Schulenberg, J., & Fuligni, A. (1993). Living arrangements and parent-adolescent relationships during the college years. *Journal of Youth and Adolescence, 22,* 171–189.

16. Sherrod, L. R., Haggerty, R. J., & Featherman, D. L. (1993). Introduction: Late adolescence and the transition to adulthood. *Journal of Research on Adolescence, 3,* 217–226.

17. U.S. Department of Commerce. Bureau of the Census. (1995). *Statistical abstract of the United States.* Washington, DC: U.S. Government Printing Office; U.S. Department of Commerce. Bureau of the Census. (2000). *Historical statistics of the United States.* Washington, DC: U.S. Government Printing Office.

18. Compas, B. E., Wagner, B. M., Slavin, L. A., & Vannatta, K. (1986). A prospective study of life events, social support, and psychological symptomology during the transition from high school to college. *American Journal of Community Psychology, 14,* 241–257; Schulenberg, J., & Maggs, J. L. (2000). *A developmental perspective on alcohol use and heavy drinking during adolescence and the transition to young adulthood.* Ann Arbor, MI: National Institute of Alcohol Addiction and Abuse.

NEW DIRECTIONS FOR YOUTH DEVELOPMENT • DOI: 10.1002/yd

19. Tinto, V. (1998). Colleges as communities: Taking research on student persistence seriously. *Review of Higher Education, 21*(2), 167–177; Roberts, S. J., & Rosenwald, G. (2001). Ever upward and no turning back: Social mobility and identity formation among first-generation college students. In D. P. McAdams, R. Josselson, & A. Lieblich (Eds.), *Turns in the road: Narrative studies of lives in transition* (pp. 91–119). Washington, DC: American Psychological Association.

20. Furstenberg. (2005).

21. Springer, L., Terenzini, P. T., Pascarella, E. T., & Nora, A. (1995). Influences on college students' orientations toward learning for self understanding. *Journal of College Student Development, 36*(1), 5–18.

22. Sherrod. (1993).

23. Furstenberg. (2005).

24. Furstenberg. (2005).

25. Roberts, R. E., & Bengton, V. L. (1996). Affective ties to parents in early adulthood and self-esteem across 20 years. *Social Psychology Quarterly, 59*, 96–106.

26. Collins, W. A. (1990). Parent-child relationships in the transition to adolescence: Continuity and change in interaction, affect, and cognition. In R. Montemayor, G. R. Adams, & T. P. Gullotta (Eds.), *From childhood to adolescence: A transitional period* (pp. 85–106). Thousand Oaks, CA: Sage; Smetana, J. G., Yau, J., & Hanson, S. (1991). Conflict resolution in families with adolescents. *Journal of Research on Adolescence, 1*, 189–206.

27. Settersten, R. A. (2005). Social policy and the transition to adulthood: Toward stronger institutions and individual capacities. In R. A. Settersten, F. Furstenberg, & R. G. Rumbaut (Eds.), *On the frontier of adulthood: Theory, research, and public policy* (pp. 534–560). Chicago: University of Chicago Press.

28. Federal Interagency Forum on Child and Family Statistics. (2000). *America's children: Key national indicators of well-being, 2000.* Washington, DC: U.S. Government Printing Office.

29. Eccles, J. S., & Barber, B. L. (1999). Student council, volunteering, basketball, or marching band: What kind of extracurricular involvement matters? *Journal of Adolescent Research, 14*, 10–43; Youniss, J., McLellan, J. A., & Yates, M. (1997). What we know about engendering civic identity. *American Behavioral Scientist, 40*, 620–631.

30. Savin-Williams, R. C., & Berndt, T. (1990). Friendships and peer relations during adolescence. In S. S. Feldman & G. R. Elliot (Eds.), *At the threshold: The developing adolescent.* Palo Alto, CA: Stanford University Press.

31. Eccles. (2002).

32. Levesque, R.J.R. (1993). The romantic experience of adolescents in satisfying love relationships. *Journal of Youth and Adolescence, 22*, 219–251; Masten, A. S., Coatsworth, J. D., Neemann, J., Gest, S. D., Tellegen, A., & Garmezy, N. (1995). The structure and coherence of competence from childhood through adolescence. *Child Development, 66*, 1635–1659; Collins, W. A. (2003). More than myth: The developmental significance of romantic relationships during adolescence. *Journal of Research on Adolescence, 13*(1), 1–24.

33. Blum, R. W., Beuhring, T., & Rinehart, P. M. (2000). *Protecting teens: Beyond race, income and family structure.* Minneapolis: Center for Adolescent Health, University of Minnesota.

34. Eccles. (2002).

35. Harter, S. (1998). The development of self-representations. In W. Damon & N. Eisenberg (Eds.), *Handbook of child psychology: Social, emotional, and personality development* (5th ed., pp. 553–618). Hoboken, NJ: Wiley; Bandura, A. (1994). *Self-efficacy: The exercise of control.* New York: Freeman; Lerner, R. M., & Galambos, N. L. (1998). Adolescent development: Challenges and opportunities for research, programs, and policies. *Annual Review of Psychology, 49,* 413–446; Deci, E. L., & Ryan, R. M. (1985). *Intrinsic motivation and self-determination in human behavior.* New York: Plenum Press.

36. Murnane, R. J., & Levy, F. (1996). *Teaching the new basic skills: Principles for educating children to thrive in a changing economy.* New York: Free Press.

37. Eccles & Gootman. (2002).

38. Eccles & Gootman. (2002).

39. Kirby, D., & Coyle, K. (1997). Youth development programs. *Children and Youth Services Review, 19*(5/6), 437–454.

40. Brown, B. B. (1990). Peer groups and peer cultures. In S. S. Feldman & G. R. Elliot (Eds.), *At the threshold: The developing adolescent* (pp. 171–196). Cambridge, MA: Harvard University Press; Ruben, K. H., Bukowski, W., & Parker, J. G. (1998). Peer interactions, relationships, and groups. In W. Damon & N. Eisenberg (Eds.), *Handbook of child psychology: Social, emotional, and personality development* (5th ed., pp. 619–700). Hoboken, NJ: Wiley.

41. Eccles & Gootman. (2002).

NICOLE ZARRETT *is a doctoral student of developmental psychology at the University of Michigan.*

JACQUELYNNE ECCLES *is Wilbert McKeachie Professor of Psychology, Women's Studies, and Education and a research scientist at the Institute for Social Research at the University of Michigan.*

If prevention programs are going to be effective in appealing to the sensibilities of urban youth and ultimately alter their behavior, they need to place diversity with respect to culture, class, and environment at the center of prevention efforts.

2

Designing for diversity: Incorporating cultural competence in prevention programs for urban youth

Marion J. Goldstein, Pedro A. Noguera

LOW-INCOME URBAN YOUTH of color frequently confront a wide variety of challenges and hardships that other young people do not experience. They are more likely to drop out of high school,[1] more likely to be unemployed,[2] more likely to experience poverty and be denied access to basic social services,[3] and more likely to become pregnant during adolescence.[4] These intensifying challenges come at a time when minority and foreign-born populations constitute the fastest-growing segment of the school-age population.[5] Census projections indicate that these populations will continue to expand due to the ongoing influx of immigrants, with the largest numbers arriving from Mexico, Asia, and Latin America.

The prevalence of hardships that urban youth of color face has contributed to the notion that this group is by its very nature at risk, and promotes stereotypes depicting these youth as irresponsible, antisocial, and even dangerous. In some cases, social scientists have

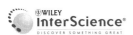

NEW DIRECTIONS FOR YOUTH DEVELOPMENT, NO. 111, FALL 2006 © WILEY PERIODICALS, INC.
Published online in Wiley InterScience (www.interscience.wiley.com) • DOI: 10.1002/yd.180
29

contributed to this discourse by suggesting that urban youth are products of a pathological "culture of poverty" that renders them incapable of overcoming environmental hardships.[6] Wide acceptance of such views among policymakers and the media has given rise to a broad set of punitive policies aimed at controlling the behavior of urban youth through security, law enforcement, and incarceration.[7]

A more positive approach to helping urban youth avoid high-risk behaviors is engaging them in prevention programs. Although some programs are successful, many are not effective in reaching diverse urban youth. In this chapter, we focus on the delivery of substance abuse prevention programs and offer an alternative program strategy— one that places diversity with respect to culture, class, and environment at the center of prevention efforts. Such an approach, we argue, is effective not only in appealing to the sensibilities of urban youth but also in altering their behavior. We believe that the core principles of this strategy are appropriate for many programs hoping to engage and have a positive impact on the lives of low-income youth of color.

About substance abuse and prevention

For most individuals, initiation into drug and alcohol use occurs during adolescence or early adulthood.[8] For many, early use is little more than a form of experimentation, but for a small but significant segment of the population, early use is the start to a long-term pattern of substance abuse. Understanding what might be done to reduce and prevent substance abuse among adolescents is increasingly recognized as an essential component of any comprehensive national prevention strategy.

Although the potential benefits of these programs are clear, many schools and community-based initiatives to curtail drug and alcohol use are ineffective because they are not tailored to meet the cultural sensibilities of diverse adolescent populations.[9] The messages and strategies adopted by most prevention programs have been designed for a white, middle-class recipient population and often are not effective in reaching student populations that are diverse with respect to race, language, culture, and socioeconomic status. Kumpfer, Alvarado, Smith, and Bellamy explain why cultural mismatch is endemic to the design of many prevention programs: "The theoretical constructs, definitions of protective or risk factors, appropriate interventions of strategies, and research evaluation strategies have all been influenced by mainstream American values."[10]

This chapter draws on the findings from research we have conducted in an urban high school located in the center of a large metropolitan area. The student population at the school was 96.9 percent nonwhite. More than two-thirds of the students were either first- or second-generation immigrants; 8.5 percent had come to the United States within the past three years. In addition, more than two-thirds came from homes where English was not the language spoken. Despite the diversity of the student population, educators at the school implemented a standard mainstream substance abuse prevention program that was being used with high school students throughout the country.

The goals of our research were to illuminate why such approaches to substance abuse prevention may be ineffective, as well as to make the case for greater attention to the need for cultural tailoring in the materials and approaches used with diverse student populations. We thus describe the concepts of cultural tailoring in the context of prevention programs. Throughout our discussion, we offer recommendations we believe will be useful to prevention programs and other programs seeking to engage and improve the outcomes for low-income youth of color.

Cultural tailoring: Surface level

Research has shown that cultural tailoring must be reflected in the surface structure of a prevention program so that interventions are matched to the observable social and behavioral characteristics of the target groups.[11] According to Pasick, D'Onofrio, and Otero-Sabogal, cultural tailoring is "the process of creating culturally sensitive interventions, often involving the adaptation of existing materials and programs for racial/ethnic populations."[12] Cultural tailoring is a strategy that has been used to enhance the cultural relevance of educational materials in order to heighten receptivity to prevention messages. Without cultural tailoring, Castro and Alarcon warn, the messages of a prevention program may be ineffective for diverse groups of learners.[13]

Successful cultural tailoring results in surface structures that are more likely to increase receptivity, comprehension, and acceptance of messages.[14] A critical component of surface-level cultural tailoring is to provide instruction and information in a language and idiom that recipients understand. This entails more than merely translating text-based information. It may also require that materials be modified in ways that are appealing and relevant to the cultural codes and social norms of adolescents. At the school where our research was conducted, 17.1 percent of students were identified as English Language Learners, but remarkably, prevention materials were available only in English.

Surface tailoring requires more than an understanding of the heritage and language of the target population. It is equally important that an understanding of students' daily lives—the challenges they face outside school, the way they interact within school, and their typical patterns of behavior—be incorporated into program design and into the training of those who will implement the prevention program. For substance abuse prevention, this also entails knowing the types of alcohol or drugs commonly used by the student population.

Surface tailoring should also recognize typical concerns of a target recipient group. For high school students, daily concerns often relate to social pressures; alcohol and drug use may be driven by peer pressure and a desire to fit in. For example, Velez and Ungemack found that peer modeling was the strongest predictor of drug involvement among Puerto Rican youth.[15] To minimize substance use risks, a prevention program must encourage students to talk about pressures they perceive in their environment and the ways in which patterns of substance use may be normalized within their environment. Such conversations are essential to facilitate the development of refusal skills and resiliency that enable students to resist perceived peer pressure. Because different ethnic/racial groups may have different perceptions of peer pressure and different methods to deal with social influences, a prevention program must be adaptive to accommodate diverse student needs.

In economically depressed areas, students may experience pressure to sell drugs as a source of income. Research has shown that where poverty is concentrated and options for employment are limited, the lure of drug trafficking may be powerful and difficult to resist.[16] In such areas, the informal sector of the economy where illegal transactions in goods and services occur may provide a greater portion of the income to residents than the formal, legal sector.[17] Under these circumstances, prevention campaigns that encourage young people to "just say no," or even the threat of long prison sentences for dealers, may not be enough to deter young people from entering the drug trade. To succeed in preventing young people from selling drugs, prevention programs may also have to address the pressures students face and the economic incentives that make it attractive.

Finally, research suggests that efforts to culturally tailor a prevention program with respect to its surface structure should incorporate members of the recipient group in program planning, development, and delivery. Hecht et al. found that minority youth were more responsive to programs in which their input was encouraged.[18] They also tended to respond favorably to teachers delivering the prevention program who were familiar with the challenges they faced in their community or were members of their own ethnic/racial group.

Cultural tailoring: Deep level

Research has shown that cultural tailoring must also entail deep-level program adaptations, which reflect how cultural, social, psychological, environmental, and historical factors influence an individual's health behaviors.[19] As with surface structure, there are several ways to make a substance abuse prevention program culturally relevant at the deep structural level. Stemming from her research involving Vietnamese, Cambodian, and Hmong refugees,

Frye recommends integrating cultural themes into health promotion messages and strategies.[20] Specifically, Frye found that kinship solidarity and the search for equilibrium were dominant cultural themes that could be linked with health messages. In a similar vein, Gloria and Peregoy found that salient Latino values such as *simpatia* (sympathy), *personalismo* (personalism), *familismo* (familial ties), *machismo* (masculinity) and *hembrismo* (brotherhood), *verguenza* (pride), and *espiritismo* (spiritualism) could be incorporated into the structure of prevention programs.[21] Finally, Wong and Piran found that in contrast to the Western culture's emphasis on the need to be independent and develop an internal locus of control, Chinese culture stresses interdependence, collectivity, and an external locus.[22] Such findings suggest that programs that reflect recognition of students' cultural values, norms, and sensibilities can increase the receptivity of adolescents to underlying prevention messages.

To accomplish deep structural tailoring, research suggests that program implementers acknowledge differences in attitudes toward substance use among and between ethnically/racially diverse student groups. Research has identified consistent correlations between one's cultural identification and his or her perspectives on health issues, receptivity to messages, and substance use behaviors. Orlandi explains, "An ethnic or racial group's shared norms, beliefs, and expectations regarding alcohol and its effects shape the group members' drinking habits, the ways in which the members behave while drinking, and their perceptions of personal and collective responsibility for the outcomes of drinking."[23]

Attitudes toward illicit drug use also tend to vary across cultures in predictable ways. Indian culture, for example, considers drug use a moral problem that brings dishonor to one's community and can cause a family to lose prestige and pride.[24] In Haiti and Cambodia, however, some narcotics are used for medicinal purposes.[25] This practice may cause some immigrants from these countries to be more accepting of drug use in some circumstances. In addition, it has been known for many years that there is variance in the age at which adolescents may be regarded as adults and allowed to make independent decisions about issues such as marriage, childbirth, and the use of controlled substances.[26] Attention to cultural perspectives and norms increases the likelihood that students will be receptive to a program's messages.

Deep-level cultural tailoring also requires an understanding of students' family child-rearing norms, which also have been found to vary across cultures. Shakib et al. explain that there is ethnic variation in parenting characteristics and child-rearing practices, including parental expectations of the parent-child relationship, reliance on authority and control, discipline, and parental monitoring.[27] Relative to middle-class and affluent whites, research has found that African Americans, Hispanics, and working-class whites are more likely to exhibit authoritative parenting styles.[28] Catalano et al. found that African American parents tend to be proactive in setting rules and monitoring their child's behavior during preadolescence, but tend to lessen the exercise of authority over their children as they grow older.[29] This type of monitoring has been found to be a protective factor that prevents early substance use initiation, but it is less effective at deterring use during the riskier teen years.

In addition, factors related to immigration and the subsequent process of assimilation and acculturation have been linked to increased risk of substance abuse and should therefore be reflected in the deep-structural tailoring of a prevention program. Research has found that as acculturation progresses with greater exposure to the cultural norms prevalent in the United States, immigrant youth experience a noticeable decline in overall health and well-being and a greater propensity to engage in a variety of risk behaviors. Similarly, a study described by Velez and Ungemack showed that drug use systematically increased with the number of years in which immigrants reported living in New York City.[30] Finally, a study by the Substance Abuse and Mental Health Services Administration revealed that although recent immigrants were less likely to engage in substance use than the U.S.-born population, immigrants who had been in the United States for ten years or longer reported drug use that was not significantly different from that of the native population.[31] This research suggests that the vulnerability of adolescent immigrants may be directly related to the stress resulting from acculturation to new societal norms, as well as to the concomitant transformation in social identity that adolescents experience during this period. Blake, Ledsky, Goodenow, and O'Donnell remind us that "as immigrants acculturate, they adopt norms, health, and risk behaviors of their immediate social reference groups and racial/ethnic peers."[32]

For all of the reasons cited, the literature suggests that a culturally competent substance abuse prevention program requires educators to have a thorough grasp of the language, values, belief systems, and challenges faced by the targeted recipient population. One may argue that it would be impossible for one program to reflect the unique cultural perspective of each student in highly diverse environments. However, Hecht et al. found that programs do not need to be narrowly tailored for each cultural or ethnic group.[33] Rather, they should incorporate a representative level of relevant cultural elements and draw on images and themes from popular culture that are likely to resonate with a wide variety of young people. By offering a broad range of culturally relevant material and allowing students to bring their own cultural perspectives into group discussions, a program can achieve cultural competency.

Implications and conclusion

Our research findings have potential implications for improving prevention programs, some of which may be of value to programs seeking to serve the needs of urban youth of color. To minimize students' risks, prevention programs should devote increased attention to informing students about the actual prevalence of adolescent substance use, which is lower than students typically perceive. Furthermore, programs should acknowledge potential ethnic/racial differences in students' perceptions about peer substance use. Our study found that African American and U.S.-born students had higher estimates of peer drug use relative to other student groups. Because adolescents tend to conform to what they perceive to be normal peer behavior,[34] these higher estimates of peer substance use may indicate that these student groups are at a heightened risk for using substances.

In our study, immigrant students had lower-frequency estimates of peer drug use relative to U.S.-born students. It is possible that with increased time in the United States, immigrant youth's social norms perceptions will become more closely matched to those reported by U.S.-born students. Over time, these changes may result in actual substance use increases among the immigrant student groups. To combat this risk, prevention programs should take advantage of the window of opportunity when immigrants are highly receptive to prevention education.[35] Specifically, prevention programs may benefit from promoting resiliency and refusal skills among immigrant youth. Such skills may help these students resist perceived peer pressure during the acculturation process, a period during which Bhattacharya and other researchers revealed that immigrants often initiate substance use.[36]

Findings from our study suggest that youth tend to overestimate the prevalence of substance use and the social pressures to engage in substance use. To help correct these misperceptions, prevention programs should encourage students to communicate with each other openly in facilitated workshops about pressures that exist within their environment. The availability of positive peer role models may provide students with the opportunity to disengage from a peer cluster that may put them at high risk for substance abuse. An obvious way a school can foster student communication is by engaging students in program development and implementation. Research attests to the success of peer-based strategies.[37]

Developing strategies to better integrate the realities that low-income urban youth of color face into prevention and youth development programs is essential to effectively offsetting the wide variety of risks they face. As suggested by our study as well as previous research, prevention initiatives are more likely to be effective if they take diversity with respect to language, culture, class, and environment into account throughout program development and implementation. Although such programs are unlikely to counter the structural factors that place large numbers of urban youth at risk (economic marginalization, housing, and job shortages, for example), they can help in promoting resilience and relief from some of the hardships urban youth endure.

Notes

1. Orfield, G., Losen, D., Wald, J., & Swanson, C. B. (2004). *Losing our future: How minority youth are being left behind by the graduation rate crisis.* Cambridge, MA: Harvard University Civil Rights Project.

2. Danziger, S. H., Sandefur, G. D., & Weinberg, D. H. (Eds.). (1994). *Confronting poverty: Prescriptions for change.* New York: Russell Sage Foundation, and Cambridge, MA: Harvard University Press.

3. Rothstein, R. (2004). *Class and schools: Using social, economic and educational reform to close the black-white achievement gap.* New York: Teachers College Press, and Washington, DC: Economic Policy Institute.

4. Luker, K. (1996). *Dubious conceptions: The politics of teenage pregnancy.* Cambridge, MA: Harvard University Press.

5. Suárez-Orozco, C., & Suárez-Orozco, M. (2001). *Children of immigration.* Cambridge, MA: Harvard University Press.

6. Murray, C. (1984). *Losing ground.* New York: Basic Books.

7. Polakow, V. (Ed.). (2001). *Violence in children's lives.* New York: Teachers College Press.

8. Kandel, D. B., & Logan, J. A. (1984). Patterns of drug use from adolescence to young adulthood: I. Periods of risk for initiation, continued use, and discontinuation. *American Journal of Public Health, 74,* 660–666.

9. Terrell, D. M. (1993). Ethnocultural factors and substance abuse: Toward culturally sensitive treatment models. *Psychology of Addictive Behaviors, 7*(3), 162–167.

10. Kumpfer, K. L., Alvarado, R., Smith, P., & Bellamy, N. (2002). Cultural sensitivity and adaptation in family-based prevention interventions. *Prevention Science, 3*(3), 241–246.

11. Rensnicow, K., Soler, R., Braithwaite, R. L., Ahluwalia, J. S., & Butler, J. (2000). Cultural sensitivity in substance use prevention. *Journal of Community Psychology, 28*(3), 271–290.

12. Pasick, R. J., D'Onofrio, C. N., & Otero-Sabogal, R. (1996). Similarities and differences across cultures: Questions to inform a third generation for health promotion research. *Health Education Quarterly, 23*(Suppl.), 142–161.

13. Castro, F. G., & Alarcon, E. (2002). Integrating cultural variables into drug abuse prevention and treatment with racial/ethnic minorities. *Journal of Drug Issues, 32*(3), 783–810.

14. Rensnicow et al. (2000).

15. Velez, C. N., & Ungemack, J. A. (1995). Psychosocial correlates of drug use among Puerto Rican youth: Generational status differences. *Social Science and Medicine, 40*(1), 91–103.

16. Wilson, W. J. (1987). *The truly disadvantaged: The inner city, the underclass, and public policy.* Chicago: University of Chicago Press.

17. Skolnick, J., & Currie, E. (1994). *Crisis in American institutions.* New York: HarperCollins.

18. Hecht, M. L., Marsiglia, F. F., Elek, E., Wagstaff, D. A., Kulis, S., & Dustman, P. (2003). Culturally grounded substance use prevention: An evaluation of the Keepin' It R.E.A.L. curriculum. *Prevention Science, 4*(4), 233–248.

19. Rensnicow et al. (2000).

20. Frye, B. A. (1995). Use of cultural themes in promoting health among Southeast Asian refugees. *American Journal of Health Promotion, 9*(4), 269–280.

21. Gloria, A. M., & Peregoy, J. J. (1996). Counseling Latino alcohol and other substance users/abusers: Cultural considerations for counselors. *Journal of Substance Abuse Treatment, 13*(2), 119–126.

22. Wong, O.N.M., & Piran, N. (1995). Western biases and assumptions as impediments in counseling traditional Chinese clients. *Canadian Journal of Counseling, 29*, 107–119.

23. Orlandi, M. A. (1992). The challenge of evaluating community-based prevention programs: A cross-cultural perspective. In M. A. Orlandi, R. Weston, & L. G. Epstein (Eds.), *Cultural competence for evaluators: A guide for alcohol and other drug abuse prevention practitioners working with ethnic/racial communities.* Washington, DC: Office for Substance Abuse Prevention, U.S. Department of Health and Human Services.

24. Bhattacharya, G. (2002). Drug abuse risks for acculturating immigrant adolescents: A case study of Asian-Indians in the United States. *Health and Social Work, 27*(3), 175–183.

25. Amodeo, M., & Jones, L. K. (1997). Viewing alcohol and other drug use cross-culturally: A cultural framework for clinical practice. *Families in Society: The Journal of Contemporary Human Services, 78*(3), 240–254.

26. Findsen, B. (2003). Older adults' communities of learning and practice. In *Proceedings of the 43rd National Conference of Adult Learning in Sydney, Australia.* Retrieved June 24, 2005, from www.ala.asn.au/conf/2003/findsen.pdf.

27. Shakib, S., Mouttapa, M., Johnson, C. A., Ritt-Olson, A., Trinidad, D. R., Gallaher, P. E., & Unger, J. B. (2003). Ethnic variation in parenting characteristics and adolescent smoking. *Journal of Adolescent Health, 33*(2), 88–97.

28. Shakib et al. (2003).

29. Catalano, R. F., Morrison, D. M., Wells, E. A., Gillmore, M. R., Iritani, B., & Hawkins, J. D. (1992). Ethnic differences in family factors related to early drug initiation. *Journal of Studies on Alcohol, 53*(3), 208–217.

30. Velez & Ungemack. (1995).

31. SAMHSA News. (2004, January/February). Acculturation increases risk for substance use by foreign-born youth. *SAMHSA News, 12*(1). Retrieved November 3, 2004, from http://www.samhsa.gov/samhsa_news/VolumeXII_1/article2.htm.

32. Blake, S. M., Ledsky, R., Goodenow, C., & O'Donnell, L. (2001). Recency of immigration, substance use, and sexual behavior among Massachusetts adolescents. *American Journal of Public Health, 91*(5), 794–798.

33. Hecht et al. (2003).

34. Stacy, A. W., Sussman, S., Dent, C. W., Burton, D., & Flay, B. R. (1992). Moderators of peer social influence in adolescent smoking. *Personality and Social Psychology Bulletin, 18*, 163–172; Musher-Eizenman, D. R., Holub, S. C., & Arnett, M. (2003). Attitude and peer influences on adolescent substance abuse: The moderating effect of age, sex and substance. *Journal of Drug Education, 33*(1), 1–23.

35. Blake, S. M., Ledsky, R., Goodenow, C., & O'Donnell, L. (2001). Receipt of school health education and school health services among adolescent immigrants in Massachusetts. *Journal of School Health, 71*(3), 105–113.

36. Bhattacharya. (2002).

37. Tobler, N. (1986). Meta-analysis of 143 adolescent drug prevention programs: Quantitative outcomes results of program participants compared to a control or comparison group. *Journal of Drug Issues, 16*(4), 537–567.

MARION J. GOLDSTEIN *is a doctoral candidate in communication and education at Teachers College, Columbia University.*

PEDRO A. NOGUERA *is a professor in the Steinhardt School of Education at New York University.*

We must prioritize the integration of technology skill building into youth development experiences in order to better prepare older youth for the challenges and responsibilities ahead.

3

Teens and technology: Preparing for the future

Georgia Hall

IN THE PAST TWO DECADES, economic, technological, demographic, and political forces have stimulated major change in the learning and working landscape for young people. Understanding how to use computers and other technology for learning, productivity, and performance has become as fundamental to a person's ability to navigate through school and career as traditional skills like reading, writing, and arithmetic.[1] The Partnership for 21st Century Skills notes that in order to thrive in the world today, young people need higher-end skills, such as the ability to communicate effectively beyond their peer groups, analyze complex information from multiple sources, write or present well-reasoned arguments, and develop solutions to interdisciplinary problems.[2] They must be prepared to spend their adult lives in a multitasking, multifaceted,

Parts of this chapter appear in Hall, G., & Israel, L. (2004). *Using technology to support academic achievement for at-risk teens during out-of-school time.* Report for the America Connects Consortium of the U.S. Department of Education. Wellesley, MA: National Institute on Out-of-School Time.

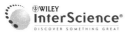

technology-driven, diverse workforce environment, and they must be equipped to do so.[3]

Skill demands have been rising, and there is every indication that this trend will continue for the foreseeable future. The disappearance of clerical and blue-collar jobs from the lower middle of the pay distribution illustrates this pattern of limited job options. People who lack the right skills drop down to compete with unskilled workers at declining wages. There are increasingly fewer positions available to workers with minimal skills. By contrast, there are more opportunities for highly skilled workers.[4] "As informational technology becomes more important for economic success and societal well-being," the possibility of being left behind becomes a strong reality.[5] These circumstances compel us to prioritize the integration of technology skill building into youth development experiences or risk the opportunity for youth to develop meaningful and productive lives.

Technology in fact is both a focus for skill and competency development and a tool for facilitating learning. As we consider approaches to integrating twenty-first-century skills into the youth development experiences for older youth, it is important to recognize the gender and race differences in technology access and use. Understanding these differences will contribute to the development and implementation of appropriate youth service strategies around technology integration. In addition, this chapter examines the particular challenges that at-risk teens face and the possible learning resource role that technology may play. Finally, this chapter proposes several approaches for integrating technology into youth development experiences.

Gender differences in computer and Internet use among teens

Several studies have shown that teenage girls tend to view the computer as a tool and a means to an end.[6] Males, in contrast, are more likely to view computers as toys or extensions of the self.[7] Young reported that males prefer computer instruction that focuses on programming, whereas females prefer computer instruction that focuses on applications.[8]

Teen females are also more practical and instrumental in their approach to computers compared to male users, who tend to use a more exploratory approach.[9] When working on computers, teenage girls generally prefer to sit down and accomplish a specific task rather than explore technological possibilities.[10]

Teenage males spend more of their out-of-school time each day on computers than their female peers.[11] Over the past fifteen years, studies have shown that males tend to seek out more extracurricular training in computer technology than females do.[12] In addition, starting in middle school, and sometimes even earlier, males tend to be more represented in after-school computer clubs.[13]

Since males typically have more out-of-school-time experiences with computers, they exhibit higher self-confidence and more positive attitudes about technology than girls do.[14] Even the most highly skilled females with significant experience in technology generally exhibit less confidence than equivalently or less-skilled male peers.[15]

While teen females tend to have more computer experience in word processing, males tend to use computers more for programming and playing games.[16] Lupart and Rabasca both reported that teen girls generally use computers for communication activities such as e-mail or visiting chatrooms.[17] They tend to dislike the narrow focus of programming courses and instead are more likely to master applications, such as databases, page layout programs, and graphics, rather than technology skills, such as programming and technological problem solving.[18]

Some research has shown that although there is no longer a gender gap in online access between males and females, there are still gender differences regarding frequency of Internet use.[19] Females tend to access the Internet less frequently, and when they are online, they generally remain there for a shorter duration.[20] Teen males are more likely than their female peers to use the Internet for surfing purposes.[21]

Research by Pinkard examined the possibility of males' and females' being attracted to games that they perceived to be geared more toward their gender-specific interests. This research questioned whether adolescent males would be more interested in computer games that were packaged and designed with their interests in mind. Her findings showed that both males and females tend to view software programs as specifically designed for males or females, but not both. Pinkard also found that both males and females are more likely to select software that they believe has been designed specifically for their gender, limiting their use and exploration of other forms of technology.[22]

The Internet, computer programs, and software all tend to feature male characters and male activities, which tend to be less engaging for females.[23] Gender-neutral software may help females overcome their reservations about exploring technology.[24]

Computers are not inherently gender biased. It is primarily the attitudinal, social, and environmental factors that play a role in the gender differences that contribute to differences in computer use.[25] Lack of role models for females in the field of computer science, as well as the differences in learning styles of males and females, contributes to gender differences in technology use. Recent research has shown there is still a difference in the amount of access males and females have to all types of technology, which affects their differences in use of and interest in computers and technology.[26] Such information can be useful in planning youth services content and delivery.

Race differences in technology use among teens

It has become increasingly clear over the past decade that race intertwines in complex ways with technological access and use. The term *digital divide* has been used to express the difference in technology access and use based on ethnicity or socioeconomic status. The digital divide has been a well-researched topic and of great national interest, prompting studies that substantively examine the challenges of and strategies for closing the digital divide in schools and communities and bringing all Americans into the digital age.

NEW DIRECTIONS FOR YOUTH DEVELOPMENT • DOI: 10.1002/yd

Technological fluency is not a skill arena in which all teens are participating equally.[27] Research has shown that access to technology is influenced by a user's assets, such as education and family background.[28]

Studies looking specifically at students from various racial backgrounds and their use of technology showed substantial differences in technology access and ownership. In a survey of students by Hoffman and Novak, 73 percent of the white students but only 32 percent of African American students owned a computer.[29] Surveys show that students who live or attend schools in low-income areas are least likely to receive full benefits from the use of educational technology.[30] Coley, Cradler, and Engel reported that students who attend schools with inadequate resources and those highly populated by minority youth have less access to most types of technology.[31]

An examination of college-bound high school seniors showed that students from minority groups were less likely to have taken word processing or computer literacy courses. Minority students were also less likely to have used a computer for English classes or for solving problems in math courses.[32]

Implications for practice

There are two important implications for program and instructional design from these findings on race and gender differences in technology use. The first is that lack of technology access influences engagement and participation choices. Teens who are already at risk of failing school due to economic, social, and educational barriers may also be marginalized from the full use of technology because of gender or race. Teens with little experience in using technology may be less likely to engage in learning tasks that rely on technological skills and experience. They may also be less attracted to programs and career pathways highlighting technology experience, expecting that such would be a mismatch to their interests or background.

A second implication is that the disparity in technological skills and experiences warrants strong consideration of youth development programs as a desirable venue for technology experiences, since the youth who have fewer technology opportunities are the same ones most often served by out-of-school-time programs. Also, budget cuts and time constraints, coupled with an intensive emphasis in schools on improving English language arts and mathematics, have relegated other subjects and skills, including technology skills, to the margins. Out-of-school-time hours may be a critical period for young people to access and engage in technology-focused experiences.[33]

At-risk teens and technology as a learning tool

Teenagers who are at high risk of failing school and often live in impoverished settings are noted in the research literature as at-risk teens. They are likely to be low achieving, of low socioeconomic status, educationally disadvantaged, academically underprepared, and English Language Learners or to have "behavior problems" or learning disabilities.[34] A report by Public/Private Ventures estimates that more than 5 million youth between the ages of fourteen and twenty-four fit this definition.[35] It is not uncommon for at-risk teens to perform below grade level, fail a grade level, or score poorly on proficiency tests.[36]

Norris proposed teaching and learning strategies that have been found to be successful with at-risk youth: (1) individualized instruction facilitated by computer-assisted instruction, (2) collaborative learning, including learning that employs computer-based simulations, computer conferencing, and database access, (3) peer tutoring, which can focus on the study of technology itself, and (4) teaching across the curriculum through computer simulations that incorporate topics in math, language arts, and science in the same lesson. Norris also explained how various uses of technology can support these four teaching strategies.[37]

Other researchers have demonstrated that technology, in a variety of forms, can have a positive influence on at-risk youth. The most effective technology strategies to support at-risk students may be those that use technology to teach "real world applications that support research, design, analysis and communication."[38]

Youth development experts agree that there are many challenges to attracting and retaining at-risk teens in out-of-school-time programs. Infusing technology-based learning strategies into programs opens up additional challenges, such as accommodating youth's learning differences, addressing youth's variations in technology approaches and experiences, providing appropriate professional development and support for instructors and activity facilitators, clarifying and connecting learning objectives and assessments, and transforming the nature of the learning environment. There is broad evidence based on the research literature that appropriate use of technology-based learning strategies can enhance the learning experience and lead to measurable academic improvements. Yet there are also implementation and utilization concerns raised about using technology as a support to academic achievement that require careful consideration when creating technology-based learning activities.

Technology and learning

The mere existence of technology-based tools in the learning environment does not guarantee that learning will transpire; the tools must be part of a "coherent education approach."[39] Goldenberg concludes that the "single most important thing that research shows is that what really matters is not the use of technology, but how it is used."[40] Research by Yegelski and Powley demonstrates that even the most basic incorporation of technology into a learning setting can encounter technological, institutional, and theoretical boundaries.[41] However, based on the volume of positive findings about the possible impacts of technology on learning while taking into consideration gender and race differences, there is sufficient reason to take advantage of the role technology can play in supporting learning for the twenty-first century.

Integrating technology skill development into youth development experiences

Youth development and out-of-school-time programs can function in ways very different from traditional classrooms, using mixed-age groups, small group learning, flexible schedules, and real-world connections. Some of these characteristics give rise to unique contexts in which young people can immerse themselves in technology skill-building activities and experiences.

Researchers contend that if program providers are to succeed with technology among teens, then content and program design must be integrated, authentic, inclusive, and self-generated. Programs that successfully integrate technology must be organic, drawing from and responding to the real lives, histories, and experiences of the youth and communities they serve.[42]

It would seem that one of the most critical roles that technology can play in supporting skill development today is to offer an attractive entry into youth development activities. Kugler notes that computer clubs are often one of the most popular out-of-school-time activities and can serve as an entry point to other learning experiences. He explains the flexibility of technology applications, suggesting that programs can use technology for remedial purposes or can design experiences that combine the development of basic skills with problem-solving exercises and opportunities for creativity.[43] Researchers suggest that applications focused on multimedia projects, which are often highly attractive to teens, can lead to success in higher-order thinking, problem solving, multistep problem solving, and synthesizing different points of view.[44]

Youth tend to be more engaged in technology-oriented programs when they are given choices in activities, when program staff provide technological support, and when they are given opportunities for reflection, discussion, and interaction.[45] In general, teens seem more attracted to approaches that attempt to infuse technology into all program activities rather than having a technology component in the program that focuses primarily on teaching technology skills.[46]

Facilitating older youth's acquisition of technology skills must continue to be a principal goal of policymakers, city leaders, and youth program providers. Research should persist in investigating strategies and learning tools that provide an "effective means of reaching essential educational objectives in the technology-driven, knowledge-based economy of this new century."[47] Supports and services need to reach out across a variety of community settings in order to ensure that all teens have access to the knowledge and skills they need to meet the demands of this century.

Notes

1. U.S. Department of Education. (1996). *Getting America's students ready for the 21st century: Meeting the technology literacy challenge: A report to the nation on technology and education.* Washington, DC: Author.

2. Partnership for 21st Century Skills. (n.d.). *The road to 21st century learning: A policymaker's guide to 21st century skills.* Washington, DC: Author.

3. Partnership for 21st Century Skills. (2004). *Learning for the 21st century: A report and mile guide for 21st century skills.* Washington, DC: Author.

4. Partnership for 21st Century Skills. (n.d.).

5. Tapscott, D. (1998). *Growing up digital: The rise of the new generation.* New York: McGraw-Hill.

6. American Association of University Women Educational Foundation Commission on Technology & Gender and Teacher Education. (2003). Girls' perspectives on the computer culture. *WEEA Digest,* 7–9, retrieved October 2006 from http://www2.edc.org/WomensEquity/pdffiles/tech_dig.pdf; American Association of University Women. (2000). *Tech-savvy: Educating girls in the new computer age.* Washington, DC: Author; Gunn, C. (1994). *Development of gender roles: Technology as an equity strategy.* Flagstaff, AZ: Center for Excellence in Education; Rabasca, L. (2000). *The Internet and computer games reinforce the gender gap.* Retrieved April 4, 2004, from http://www.apa.org/monitor/oct00/games/html.

7. American Association of University Women. (2000).

8. Young, B. (2000). Gender differences in student attitudes toward computers. *Journal of Research on Technology in Education, 33*(2), 204–216.

9. Gunn, C., French, S., McLeod, H., McSporran, M., & Conole, G. (2002). Gender issues in computer-supported learning. *Association for Learning Technology Journal, 10*(1), 32–44.

10. Koch, M. (1994). Opening up technology to both genders. *Education Digest, 60*(3), 18–23.

11. Lupart, J., & Cannon, E. (2002). Computers and career choices: Gender differences in grades 7 and 10 students. *Gender, Technology and Development, 6*(2), 233–248; Mark, J. (1992). Beyond equal access: Gender equity in learning with computers. *WEEA Digest,* 1, retrieved October 2006 from http://www2.edc.org/WomensEquity/pubs/digests/digest-beyond.html#Beyond.

12. Hess, R. D., & Miura, I. T. (1985). Gender differences in enrollment in computer camps and classes. *Sex Roles, 13*(3/4), 193–203; Lockheed, M. E.

(1985). Women, girls, and computers: A first look at evidence. *Sex Roles,* *13*(3/4), 115–122; Miura, I. T. (1986, April 16–20). *Understanding gender differences in middle school computer interest and use.* Paper presented at the Annual Meeting of the American Educational Research Association, San Francisco; Weinman, J., & Cain, L. (1999). Technology—the new gender gap. *Technos,* *8*(1), 9–12.

13. American Association of University Women. (2000); American Association of University Women. (2003); Kirkpatrick, H., & Cuban, L. (1998). Should we be worried? What the research says about gender differences in access, use, attitudes, and achievement with computers. *Educational Technology,* *38*(4), 56–61; Sanders, M. G., Allen-Jones, G. L., & Abel, Y. (2002). Involving families and communities in the education of children and youth placed at risk. In S. Stringfield & D. Land (Eds.), *Educating at-risk students* (Vol. 2). Chicago: University of Chicago Press.

14. Gunn et al. (2002); Mark. (1992); Weinman & Cain. (1999); Young. (2000).

15. Margolis, J., & Fisher, A. (2002). *Unlocking the computer clubhouse: Women in computing.* Cambridge, MA: MIT Press.

16. American Association of University Women. (2000); Lockheed. (1985); Miura. (1986); Weinman & Cain. (1999); Coley, R., Cradler, J., & Engel, P. (1998). *Computers and classrooms: The status of technology in U.S. schools.* Princeton, NJ: Educational Testing Service.

17. Lupart & Cannon. (2002); Rabasca. (2000).

18. American Association of University Women. (2000).

19. Debell, M., & Chapman, C. (2003). *Computer and Internet use by children and adolescents in 2001.* Washington, DC: U.S. Department of Education, National Center for Education Statistics; Ono, H., & Zavodny, M. (2003). Gender and the Internet. *Social Science Quarterly, 84*(1), 111–121; Young. (2000).

20. Young. (2000).

21. Lupart & Cannon. (2002).

22. Pinkard, N. (in press). *Through the eyes of gender: A formative study of how the perceived masculinity and/or femininity of software applications influence students' software preferences.* Chicago: Center for School Improvement, University of Chicago.

23. Nelson, C. S., & Watson, J. A. (1991). The computer gender gap: Children's attitudes, performance and socialization. *Journal of Educational Technology Systems, 19*(4), 345–353; Rabasca. (2000).

24. Lynn, K.-M., Raphael, C., Olefsky, K., & Bachen, C. M. (2003). Bridging the gender gap in computing: An integrative approach to content design for girls. *Journal of Educational Computing Research, 28*(2), 143–162.

25. Mark. (1992).

26. Brown, B. L. (2001). *Women and minorities in high-tech careers.* Columbus, OH: ERIC Clearinghouse on Adult, Career, and Vocational Education; Miller, L. M., Schweingruber, H., & Brandenburg, C. L. (2001). Middle school students' technology practices and preferences: Re-examining gender differences. *Journal of Educational Multimedia and Hypermedia, 10*(2), 125–140.

27. Kominski, R., & Newburger, E. C. (1999). *Access denied: Changes in computer ownership and use: 1984–1997.* Paper presented at the Annual Meeting of the American Sociological Association, Chicago.

28. Ba, H., Culp, K. M., Green, L., Henriquez, A., & Honey, M. (2001). *Effective technology use in low-income communities: Research review for the American Connects Consortium.* Newton, MA: America Connects Consortium.

29. Hoffman, D. L., & Novack, T. P. (1998). Bridging the racial divide on the Internet. *Science, 280,* 390–391.

30. Solomon, G. (2002). Digital equity: It's not just about access anymore. *Technology and Learning, 22*(9), 18–26.

31. Coley, R., Cradler, J., & Engel, P. (1998). *Computers and classrooms: The status of technology in U.S. schools.* Princeton, NJ: Educational Testing Service.

32. Coley et al. (1998).

33. California Department of Education. (2000). *Science camp: Enrichment training for school-age care.* Sacramento, CA: Author.

34. Land, D., & Legters, N. (2002). The extent and consequences of risk in U.S. education. In S. Stringfield & D. Land (Eds.), *Educating at-risk students* (Vol. 2). Chicago: University of Chicago Press; Moore, J. L., Laffey, J. M., Espinosa, L. M., & Lodree, A. W. (2002). Bridging the digital divide for at-risk students: Lessons learned. *TechTrends, 46*(2), 5–9; Page, M. S. (2002). Technology-enriched classrooms: Effects on students of low-socioeconomic status. *Journal of Research on Technology in Education, 34*(4), 389–409.

35. Public/Private Ventures. (2002). *Serving high-risk youth: Lessons from research and programming.* Philadelphia: Author.

36. Ohio State Legislative Office of Education Oversight. (1997). *Programs for at-risk high school students.* Columbus, OH: Author. (ED 416 265)

37. Norris, C. (1994). Computing and the classroom: Teaching the at-risk student. *Computing Teacher, 4,* 12–14.

38. Chavez, R. C. (1990). The development of story writing within an IBM Writing to Read Program lab among language minority students: Preliminary findings of a naturalistic study. *Computers in the Schools, 7*(1/2), 121–144; Dunkel, P. (1990). Implications of the CAI effectiveness research for limited English proficient learners. *Computers in the Schools, 7*(1/2), 23–26; Means, B. (1997). *Critical issue: Using technology to enhance engages learning for at-risk students.* Naperville, IL: North Central Regional Educational Laboratory; Merino, B. J., Legarreta, D., Coughran, C. C., & Hoskins, J. (1990). Interaction at the computer by language minority boys and girls paired with fluent English proficient peers. *Computers in the Schools, 7*(1/2), 109–119.

39. National Research Council. (2000). Technology to support learning. In J. D. Bransford, A. L. Brown, R. R. Cocking, M. S. Donovan, & J. W. Pellegrino (Eds.), *How people learn: Brain, mind, experience, and school.* Washington, DC: National Academy Press.

40. Goldenberg, E. P. (2000). *Thinking (and talking) about technology in math classrooms.* Newton, MA: Education Development Center.

41. Yagelski, R. P., & Powley, S. (1996). Virtual connections and real boundaries: Teaching writing and preparing writing teachers on the Internet. *Computers and Composition, 12,* 25–36.

42. Benton Foundation. (2003). *Preparing disadvantaged youth for the workforce of tomorrow.* Washington, DC: Author.

43. Kugler, M. R. (2001). After-school programs are making a difference. *NASSP Bulletin, 85*(626), 3–11.

44. Valdez, G., McNabb, M. L., Foertsch, M., Anderson, M., Hawkes, M., & Raack, L. (2000). *Computer-based technology and learning: Evolving uses and expectations.* Oak Brook, IL: North Central Regional Educational Library.

45. Alexander, P. A., & Wade, S. E. (2000). Contexts that promote interest, self-determination, and learning: Lasting impressions and lingering questions. *Computers in Human Behavior, 16*, 349–358.

46. California Community Technology Policy Group. (2002). *After-school and community technology agendas for youth: Preliminary thoughts about our shared interests.* Retrieved March 5, 2004, from http://www.techpolicybank.org/cctpg.html.

47. Dede, C. (2000). A new century demands new ways of learning. In D. T. Gordon (Ed.), *The digital classroom.* Cambridge, MA: Harvard Education Letter.

GEORGIA HALL *is a research scientist at the National Institute on Out-of-School Time, part of the Wellesley Centers for Women at Wellesley College.*

*Secondary schools can improve the academic
achievement of all students by using a reform framework grounded in research about how young people
develop and how schools can promote students'
engagement and learning.*

4

First Things First: A framework for successful secondary school reform

James P. Connell, Adena M. Klem

RESEARCH ON YOUTH, and specifically on economically disadvantaged youth, demonstrates the importance of educational outcomes as precursors of important life outcomes such as economic self-sufficiency, healthy family and social relationships, and good citizenship.[1]

If youth development initiatives are going to focus on outcomes that we know are important in settings that we know can change these outcomes, the first outcomes should be educational, and the first setting should be school. School reform presents the most feasible, defensible, and informed opportunity for public policy to improve the life chances of children and youth in disadvantaged communities.

Framework for school reform

The Institute for Research and Reform in Education (IRRE) is dedicated to helping schools raise the academic performance of all

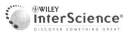

students to levels required for postsecondary education and high-quality employment. To accomplish this, IRRE developed First Things First (FTF), a reform framework grounded in research about how young people develop and how schools promote students' engagement and learning in the process. Currently FTF is operating at twenty-six high schools and forty-five middle and elementary schools in nine school districts across the country (http//www. irre.org) with the goal of improving critical student outcomes such as attendance, test scores, persistence, and graduation rates.

The FTF framework (see Figure 4.1) identifies student and school outcomes, critical features essential to improve those outcomes, specific strategies for putting the critical features in place, and structured and timed processes for planning, capacity building, and continuous improvement. In order for meaningful changes in student outcomes to occur, the framework posits that certain conditions must exist:

- A more personalized learning environment through the creation of small learning communities (SLCs)
- A partnership between the student, his or her family, and a staff person from the student's SLC who acts as an advocate for that student and family, all of whom work together to ensure the youth's success in school
- High-quality teaching and learning that is rigorous, engaging, and aligned with state standards and high-stakes assessment

Within the FTF framework are seven critical features of school reform essential for achieving improved outcomes for students and schools (see Exhibit 4.1). This chapter explores the first four critical features, which focus on students. We also introduce the three specific strategies for achieving these features.

Critical features 1 and 2: Greater continuity of care and increased instructional time

All major school reform strategies share the hypothesis that better relationships between adults and students contribute to improved

NEW DIRECTIONS FOR YOUTH DEVELOPMENT • DOI: 10.1002/yd

Figure 4.1. First Things First Framework

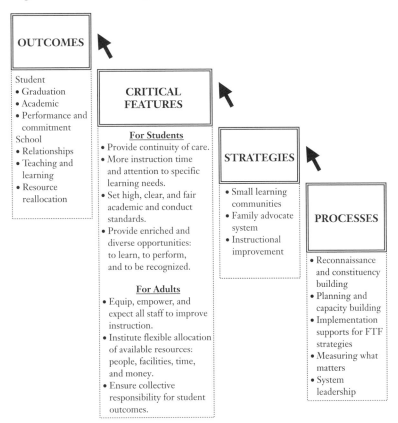

OUTCOMES

Student
• Graduation
• Academic
• Performance and
  commitment
School
• Relationships
• Teaching and
  learning
• Resource
  reallocation

CRITICAL
FEATURES

For Students
• Provide continuity of care.
• More instruction time
  and attention to specific
  learning needs.
• Set high, clear, and fair
  academic and conduct
  standards.
• Provide enriched and
  diverse opportunities:
  to learn, to perform,
  and to be recognized.

For Adults
• Equip, empower, and
  expect all staff to improve
  instruction.
• Institute flexible allocation
  of available resources:
  people, facilities, time,
  and money.
• Ensure collective
  responsibility for student
  outcomes.

STRATEGIES

• Small learning
  communities
• Family advocate
  system
• Instructional
  improvement

PROCESSES

• Reconnaissance
  and constituency
  building
• Planning and
  capacity building
• Implementation
  supports for FTF
  strategies
• Measuring what
  matters
• System
  leadership

educational outcomes for students.[2] Extensive research on children and youth in diverse educational settings supports this hypothesis.[3]

In economically disadvantaged settings, serious and deeply rooted challenges make it especially difficult to build these relationships. Gaps of class, ethnicity, and places of residence have historically separated professionals in urban schools from the students and families they serve. At the same time, these are the schools where strong ties between adults and students can make the greatest difference.

Research demonstrates that strong relationships between young people and adults are forged when the young person experiences the adult providing valuable psychological resources (time, respect,

Exhibit 4.1. Seven Critical Features of the FTF Framework

For Students

- Critical Feature 1: Provide continuity of care by forming small learning communities that keep the same group of professionals, students, and their families together for extended periods during the day and across multiple school years.
- Critical Feature 2: Provide additional instructional time and attention to individual learning needs, primarily by identifying struggling reading and math learners and redistributing time and professional staff to meet these and all learners' needs.
- Critical Feature 3: Set high, clear, and fair standards for academics and conduct, clearly defining what all students will know and be able to do by the time they leave each level of schooling (elementary, middle, and high school) and then assessing their progress at key points along the way.
- Critical Feature 4: Provide enriched and diverse opportunities: to learn, by making learning more active and connected in safe and respectful environments; to perform, by linking assessment strategies that use multiple modes of learning and performance directly to standards; and to be recognized by creating incentives for student achievement and by providing leadership opportunities in academic and non-academic areas.

For Adults

- Critical Feature 5: Equip, empower, and expect staff to implement effective instructional practices by giving teachers the authority and expertise to make effective instructional decisions through opportunities for continuous staff learning, clear expectations about what good teaching and learning look like, and strong instructional leadership at all levels to ensure all teachers meet these expectations.
- Critical Feature 6: Give small learning communities and schools the flexibility to redirect resources (time, money, people, and space) quickly to meet emerging needs.
- Critical Feature 7: Ensure collective responsibility by providing collective incentives and consequences for small learning communities, schools, and district staff, based on improvements in student performance and commitment.

caring); setting high, clear, and fair standards; and encouraging expressions of individuality.[4]

We also know that student learning benefits when students receive more adult support and guidance during instructional periods and from the same adults over longer periods of time.[5] Under these conditions, students have greater access to teachers, more individualized attention, and a better understanding of the classroom routine. At the same time, teachers are more likely to use active engagement strategies that have been linked to improvements in student performance: hands-on instructional approaches such as materials students can manipulate themselves, interest centers, and cooperative learning structures.[6]

Continuity of care

To achieve these conditions, schools need to provide greater continuity of care by keeping students with a stable group of adults across longer periods during the school day and across multiple years of their school experience. They also must extend the instructional time so that students can meet higher academic standards.

How much continuity of care is enough? Almost all exemplary schools we have observed have longer instructional periods (one to two hours) with the same teacher or groups of teachers across the school day and keep students with the same adults across multiple school years.[7] This is in contrast to the typical urban middle school in which, based on an eight-period day, students have about twenty-four teachers and change classes more than four thousand times over their three years in the school.

Going beyond the evidence, it stands to reason that students will feel more secure and be more productive when students and adults work together in small, flexible groupings that remain focused on their task for as long as they need and that remain relatively consistent over multiple years. Deborah Meier, founder of Central Park East Secondary School, points out that such arrangements are much more consistent with the nature of people's work lives beyond the school years. She asks: "When will young people ever again work for eight different bosses a day, one at a time, for forty-five minutes apiece on completely isolated sets of tasks?"[8]

Perhaps most important is continuity across school years. Achieving continuity of care across school years requires that professionals stretch the perceived boundaries of their practice. For example, former ninth-grade teachers who see their students throughout their high school careers must attend to instructional and interpersonal needs of students as they undergo the transition from their early to late teenage years. Fortunately, teachers whose small learning communities have implemented continuity of care at the elementary, middle, and high school levels report that the social and academic benefits more than offset the challenges. These benefits include:

- The efficiencies that come with knowing most students at the start of each school year
- Increased student self-confidence and social skills
- Stronger relationships with students and their families
- Increased knowledge about children's intellectual strengths and weaknesses
- The opportunity to track student progress across school years
- More opportunities to individualize learning for students[9]

Deborah Meier aptly summarizes the benefits of continuity of care: "When you have a student for a year, she is on your mind. When you have a student in your class for two to three years, she is on your conscience."[10]

Continuity of care across school and home occurs when adults from these settings form personal relationships intended to support individual students' academic achievement and commitment. These relationships can and have been formed when adults in small learning communities commit themselves to act as advocates for a group of students and their families from the time the students enter the small learning community until they successfully move on to post-secondary education or high-quality employment.[11]

Advocates act as partners with students and their families in setting academic and behavioral targets, monitoring progress on these targets, and formulating appropriate intervention strategies at home and at school to ensure students achieve their targets. When teachers take on this advocate role, parent attendance at teacher conferences and student accountability increase dramatically.[12]

Increased instructional time

Many students in urban schools need increased instructional time to meet the increasingly rigorous academic standards they face, par-

NEW DIRECTIONS FOR YOUTH DEVELOPMENT • DOI: 10.1002/yd

ticularly in language arts and math.[13] With this additional time, students without the prerequisite skills in these areas will be able to catch up without failing and having to retake courses. Students who are on track use the additional time to move to higher levels of mastery. How much additional instructional time and how often the lower student-adult ratios during this time will occur depend on the resources and priorities of the school and district.

Critical features 3 and 4: High, clear, and fair standards and enriched opportunities for students

The first two critical features (continuity of care and increased instructional time) help provide the foundation for the next two critical features, which require students to meet the challenges posed by higher standards and the new and more difficult work these standards demand.

Standards

The standards movement is visible at all levels of educational policy. Leading educational theorists,[14] practitioners,[15] advocates,[16] and policymakers[17] are making compelling arguments for the importance of high, clear, and fair academic standards for all students in urban schools.

State standards describe what students should know and be able to do, and states have developed assessments aligned with such standards.[18] While states vary greatly in their specificity, these standards typically include what students will know and be able to do at key points in elementary, middle, and high school and when they graduate from high school. When specified levels of performance on assessments reflecting these standards are fully implemented, they determine not only student graduation but also student advancement (for example, from elementary to middle to high school), course grades, and successful completion of projects or units of study within a course. These are also the standards that states expect will drive curriculum and instruction in every classroom.

In First Things First, we have expanded the critical feature of setting high, clear, and fair academic standards to include conduct standards. Developmental and educational research supports the importance of setting high standards and expectations for students' individual and social conduct. And youth development research and programs emphasize the importance of involving older children and youth in establishing, articulating, and enforcing these standards.[19]

Diverse learning opportunities

The need for standards is compelling. Equally important are more diverse opportunities for students to learn, perform, and be recognized if they are to have any real hope of achieving these standards. In fact, we believe that raising expectations and standards without enriching and diversifying students' opportunities to learn will do more harm than good. Thus, First Things First, like other reform initiatives,[20] links high academic and behavioral standards with the supports and opportunities that students need to meet them:

- More enriched and diverse opportunities to learn include more active, integrated, cooperative, and real-world learning. These opportunities have all been shown to yield higher levels of student engagement and deeper levels of student learning in diverse groups of students.[21] Student engagement in learning is also linked to less disruptive behavior and lower levels of suspensions.[22]
- Opportunities to perform include multiple and more authentic modes of assessment that are linked to content standards and that teachers use to guide instruction.[23]
- Opportunities to be recognized include formal and informal ways for students to be leaders among their peers, to have their work recognized, and to demonstrate their uniqueness as well as their collective contribution to their class, school, and community.[24]

These opportunities for students appear in all schools to some degree, but in successful schools, they are key elements in the everyday lives of all students.

Three key strategies

The critical features of FTF are implemented through three key strategies: small learning communities, a family advocate system, and instructional improvement.

Small learning communities

In FTF, small learning communities (SLCs) encompass ten to twenty staff and no more than 180 students at the elementary level and 350 students at the middle and high school levels. Students stay in their SLCs for most classes during the school day and across multiple years—for example, all four years of high school or all three years of middle school. With a relatively small number of students, each SLC is a size that allows staff to know every student personally, but still large enough to include teachers who can ensure the needed breadth of content expertise. All high school and many middle school SLCs mix grades with students from all grade levels in the building in each SLC, making it possible to base instruction and curriculum on individual academic needs and interests rather than only grade levels. SLCs are also the place where staff members study data on individual students in their SLC, take collective responsibility for every student's success, and make key decisions about discipline, staffing, time use, and budget.

All FTF high schools and many FTF middle schools have themes selected by staff, students, and community input. Several FTF schools also have transitional communities: some enable students who are over age for their grade level to recover credits rapidly and join the mainstream SLCs within a year, back on track toward graduation; others provide intensive literacy support to students with low levels of English proficiency to help them meet the challenges of the core curriculum in the mainstream SLCs.

Family advocate system

SLCs include students' families through the family advocate system. This strategy puts a school adult in the corner of every student and strengthens the kind of family involvement that is important for student achievement. Each staff member becomes an advocate for fifteen to twenty students and their families, stays with them all the years they are in the school, and does whatever it takes to help those students succeed. Family advocates contact families regularly and involve them, along with their child, in setting and meeting academic and behavioral goals. A family advocate's responsibilities include:

- Meeting with students assigned to his or her advocacy group at the beginning of the school year, get to know them as individuals, and, in high school, help each one develop an academic plan for meeting the district's graduation requirements
- Meeting with the advocacy group at least weekly during a scheduled family advocate period
- Monitoring students' progress continuously through use of the academic and behavioral profile, a summary report of student outcomes created by IRRE
- Maintaining personal contact with each student in the group throughout the year with at least a five-minute weekly check-in
- Contacting the families of his or her students at least once a month
- Holding at least two family conferences annually (one per semester) with students and their families together to build relationships with families, share information about the students' academic and behavioral progress, review existing goals, and set new goals
- Meeting regularly with SLC colleagues to share information and monitor students' academic and behavioral progress
- Acting as an advocate for their students within the SLC and school
- Referring students or families, or both, to the support services they need in the school or the community

The family advocate system plays a major role in easing the transition from elementary to middle school and from middle to high school. SLCs assign a family advocate to each new student. Many family advocates contact students' families over the summer to establish a relationship at the outset. Transitions between grade levels are eased further by the fact that the same advocate is responsible for the same group of students and their families the entire time the student is in the school. Advocates help students through the academic and social difficulties associated with being in a new school; that may mean helping the student develop the study skills to succeed with a more demanding curriculum, securing additional supports if the student's skills are below grade level, or helping the student navigate the complexities of the new social environment. Advocates at the high school level involve the SLC's guidance counselor to make sure that students develop a plan with the requisite courses for graduation and to help with applications for college or postsecondary employment.

Instructional improvement

Three overarching instructional goals have become the focus of FTF instructional improvement:

Engagement: Students actively process information (listening, reading, thinking, making) and communicate information (speaking, performing, writing) in ways that indicate they are focused on the task at hand and interested in it.

Alignment: What is being taught and what students are being asked to do are aligned with the standards and curriculum, are on time and on target with the scope and sequence of the course of study, and use methods of assessment that include those that students will encounter in high-stakes testing.

Rigor: Materials and instructional strategies challenge and encourage all students to produce work or respond at or above grade level. All students are required to demonstrate mastery at these levels and have the opportunity for reteaching to mastery.

To achieve these goals, teachers need time outside the classroom to plan together and focus on instructional improvement and the support in protecting and using this valuable time effectively. During common planning time, staff make classroom visits within and across disciplines, discuss what they see, and consider how to implement new practices in their own classrooms. They study student work together to evaluate the rigor of a particular assignment, look at the resulting student output, and talk about ways to improve it. It is also the forum for looking at student data. Since SLC members share the same students, together they set targets based on data about student performance, create action plans to meet those targets, and regularly review data to monitor progress.

Professional development opportunities allow staff to learn about new instructional strategies for strengthening student engagement, aligning instruction with state and local standards, and incorporating high expectations for all students into their lesson planning and teaching practices. Ongoing coaching and follow-up allow staff to fully integrate new strategies into their instructional repertoire.

Conclusion

The ultimate goal of the critical features in school site reform is enhanced student performance and commitment. To achieve this, these features must have enough force to dislodge the behavioral regularities and bureaucratic structures that many reform theorists argue are responsible for limiting creativity in schools and causing innovation to wither over time.[25]

Independent evaluations have now confirmed the finding that with consistent and focused supports from their districts and IRRE, schools serving large numbers of minority and economically disadvantaged students can produce exciting results that include higher persistence and graduation rates and significantly better performance on state tests.[26]

Notes

1. Gambone, M. A., Klem, A. M., & Connell, J. P. (2002). *Finding out what matters for youth: Testing key links in a community action framework for youth devel-*

opment. Philadelphia: Youth Development Strategies and the Institute for Research and Reform in Education.

2. Comer, J. P., Haynes, N. M., Joyner, E. T., & Ben-Avie, M. (Eds.). (1996). *Rallying the whole village: The Comer process for reforming education.* New York: Teachers College Press.

3. Croninger, R. G., & Lee, V. E. (2001). Social capital and dropping out of high schools: Benefits to at-risk students of teachers' support and guidance. *Teachers College Record, 103*(4), 548–581.

4. Rhodes, J., Grossman, J., & Reche, N. (2000). Agents of change: Pathways through which mentoring relationships influence adolescents' academic adjustment. *Child Development, 71,* 1662–1671.

5. Kemple, J., & Snipes, J. (2000). *Career academies: Impacts on student engagement and performance in high school.* New York: Manpower Demonstration Research Corporation.

6. Lee, C. D. (2000). Signifying in the zone of proximal development. In C. D. Lee & P. Smagorinsky (Eds.), *Vygotskian perspectives on literacy research: Constructing meaning through collaborative inquiry* (pp. 191–225). Cambridge: Cambridge University Press.

7. Legters, N. E., Balfanz, R., Jordan, W. J., & McPartland, J. M. (2002). *Comprehensive reform for urban high schools: A talent development approach.* New York: Teachers College Press.

8. Meier, D. (1995). *The power of their ideas: Lessons for America from a small school in Harlem.* Boston: Beacon Press.

9. National Middle School Association. (1997). *Exemplary middle schools.* Retrieved from http://www.nmsa.org/ressum4.htm.

10. Personal conversation between J. Connell and D. Meiers, May 20, 1995.

11. Meier, D. (1997). How our schools could be. In E. Clinchy (Ed.), *Transforming public education: A new course for America's future.* New York: Teachers College Press.

12. Meier. (1997).

13. Legters, N. E., Balfanz, R., Jordan, W. J., & McPartland, J. M. (2002). *Comprehensive reform for urban high schools: A talent development approach.* New York: Teachers College Press.

14. Comer et al. (1996).

15. American Federation of Teachers. (1999).

16. Marzano, R. J., & Kendall, J.S. (1998). *A comprehensive guide to designing standards-based districts, schools, and classrooms.* Denver, CO: Mid-Continental Regional Educational Laboratory.

17. Ravitch, D. (1995). *National standards in American education: A citizen's guide.* Washington DC: Brookings Institute.

18. Lewis, A. (1999). *1998 CRESST Conference Proceedings: Comprehensive systems for educational accounting and improvement. R&D Results.* Los Angeles: University of California, National Center for Research on Evaluation, Standards, and Student Testing and Center for the Study of Evaluation.

19. Eccles, J. S., & Gootman, J. (Eds.). (2002). *Community programs to promote youth development.* Washington, DC: National Academy Press.

20. Legters et al. (2002).

21. Langer, J. A. (2001). Beating the odds: Teaching middle and high school students to read and write well. *American Educational Research Journal, 38*(4), 837–880.

22. Marks, H. M. (2000). Student engagement in instructional activity: Patterns in the elementary, middle, and high school years. *American Educational Research Journal, 37*(1), 153–184.

23. Stipek, D. (2002). Good instruction is motivating. In A. Wigfield & J. Eccles, (Eds.), *Development of achievement motivation* (pp. 309–332). Orlando, FL: Academic Press.

24. Marzano, R. J., Pickering, D. J., & Pollock, J. E. (2001). *Classroom instruction that works: Research-based strategies for increasing student achievement.* Alexandria, VA: Association for Supervision and Curriculum Development.

25. Quartz, K. H. (1995). Sustaining new educational communities: Toward a new culture of school reform. In *Yearbook* (vol. 94, pt. 1, pp. 240–252). Chicago: National Society for the Study of Education.

26. Gambone, M. A., Klem, A. M., Summers, J. A., Akey, T., & Sipe, C. (2004). *Turning the tide: The achievements of the First Things First education reform in the Kansas City, Kansas Public School District.* Philadelphia: Youth Development Strategies. Retrieved September 7, 2005, from http///www.ydsi.org; MDRC. *Scaling up First Things First: Final report.* New York: MDRC, retrieved September 7, 2005, from http://www.mdrc.org.

JAMES P. CONNELL *is the president and cofounder of the Institute for Research and Reform in Education, Philadelphia.*

ADENA M. KLEM *is the operations manager for First Things First at the Institute for Research and Reform in Education, Philadelphia.*

Three after-school initiatives have successfully engaged large numbers of high school youth in activities to increase their school success and allow them to master and apply real world skills. Lessons learned by these afterschool pioneers can inform those interested in serving older youth after school.

5

Three high school after-school initiatives: Lessons learned

*Sarah Barr, Jennifer Birmingham,
Jennifer Fornal, Rachel Klein, Sam Piha*

LITTLE ATTENTION HAS BEEN PAID to older youth in the recent expansion of school-based after-school programs. High school clubs and community-based programs have existed for years, but many have struggled to sustain the participation of teens. Alarmed by the large numbers of high school–age youth who are disengaged at school and leaving high school without a diploma or the important skills for the workplace, policymakers and youth advocates are beginning to see high school afterschool as the new frontier in after-school programming.

Despite potential benefits of quality high school after-school programs, there is a dramatic shortage of such programs. Relatively few after-school initiatives across the country even offer

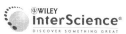

NEW DIRECTIONS FOR YOUTH DEVELOPMENT, NO. 111, FALL 2006 © WILEY PERIODICALS, INC.
Published online in Wiley InterScience (www.interscience.wiley.com) • DOI: 10.1002/yd.183

programs on high school campuses. Of those that do, many are still learning about what it takes to meet student interest and needs. This chapter reviews the insights and lessons learned from three after-school initiatives that have shown success in attracting high school students to their programs and engaging them in meaningful activities to support their success in school and transition to early adulthood.

The initiatives

The After School Safety and Education for Teens (ASSETs) initiative represents California's first attempt to direct after-school funds to serve the academic and developmental needs of high school–age youth. In 2002, the California legislature dedicated a portion of California's federal 21st Century Community Learning Center Funds to support after-school programs for high school youth. The legislation stipulated that programs be developed to "meet the needs of high school pupils through an assessment of the needs and interests of low-performing pupils, provide academic assistance to help pupils prepare for the high school exit exam, and provide enrichment activities, including, but not limited to vocational education, community service activities, and mentoring opportunities." Each ASSETs program serves up to 330 students daily, with an annual operating budget between $100,000 and $250,000. Many of the participants attend programs three to four times per week. Currently there are close to sixty after-school programs operating at low-performing high schools across California, representing an investment of $9.4 million.[1]

After School Matters (ASM) was created in 2001 to coordinate city resources and public space and expand the Gallery 37 apprenticeship model into the areas of technology, communications, sports, horticulture, and others. ASM is a nonprofit organization that partners with the City of Chicago, the Chicago Public Schools, the Chicago Park District, the Chicago Public Library, and community-based organizations to expand out-of-school opportunities for Chicago teens. ASM's predecessor, Gallery 37, was created in 1991 and paired young artists with working professional artists in an apprenticeship-like environment; teens learned skills while creating murals for public installation, offering free performances in a downtown location, and creating paintings and sculptures for sale. ASM apprenticeships are hands-on, interactive programs led by skilled professionals where teens have the opportunity to explore different career paths and develop marketable skills such as teamwork, communications, and problem solving. AFM is designed to engage teens in learning new skills within the context of their school and prepare them for the workforce that awaits them. By being school based, participants are motivated to attend school regularly. ASM works in thirty-five neighborhood clusters of schools, parks, and libraries and over 120 community-based organizations with capacity for over twenty-two thousand teens each year.

The After-School Corporation (TASC) was established in 1998 to enhance the quality and availability of free after-school programming for public school students in New York City and State. TASC provides grants, training, and technical assistance to nonprofit organizations that have partnered with a public school. After-school activities are school based, and all students in grades K–12 who are enrolled in the host school are eligible to participate. The TASC model mandates that a full-time site coordinator lead each project and participants attend regularly.

All TASC projects offer an array of academic, athletic, and arts enrichment, and projects seek to nurture healthy youth development by encouraging positive adult and peer relationships. TASC high school projects add a focus on college preparation and career training, such as TASC's Scholars and Mentors program, which trains and pays high school youth to work in TASC projects located in elementary and middle schools. In school year 2003–04, TASC funded fourteen nonprofit organizations to provide after-school services to high school students in twenty public schools. Together, these projects serve 3,920 New York City high school students.

Program evaluation: Early findings

Although there has been limited research on the impact of high school after-school programs on those who attend, both ASM in Chicago and New York City TASC formative evaluations show promising results. An interim evaluation report of California's ASSETs program, conducted by WestEd, was released in January 2006 and is available on its Web site (http://www.wested.org). The final report will be issued in 2007. Below, we review some key findings from the ASM and TASC evaluations.

School attendance

An important factor in young people's school success is school attendance. Policy Studies Associates conducted a multiyear evaluation of the TASC initiative. It found that youth with poor attendance (second-lowest quartile of school attendance) prior to joining a TASC program attended school nearly 23 more days than the nonparticipants who had similar attendance patterns the prior year. Those who attended the after-school program regularly did even better: 28.9 more days than similar peers. TASC participants who were the least engaged in school (lowest attendance quartile in the previous year) decreased their school attendance at less than half the rate of comparable nonparticipants.

Similar to the TASC study, Chapin Hall Center for Children at the University of Chicago found that teens who participated in ASM regularly (80 percent of the time) had higher school attendance than nonparticipants with similar demographics and level of school performance.

On track for graduation

The TASC evaluation found that program participants were more likely to pass selected New York Regents (high school exit) exams and were much more likely to pass five or more Regents exams than nonparticipants. Furthermore, the average number of high school credits for graduation earned by participants a year after program exposure was significantly higher than that of nonparticipants.

NEW DIRECTIONS FOR YOUTH DEVELOPMENT • DOI: 10.1002/yd

Skills for living and working

Robert Halpern, of the Erikson Institute, conducted an observational study of the ASM apprenticeship model.[2] In his observation, he points to many ways in which the ASM model helps teens learn new skills and become engaged in their schoolwork and their future. He observed that because the program was product based and established a worklike setting, youth developed important life skills and perspectives that will assist them as they make the transition out of school into the larger world. These life skills include the ability to work productively within a team, assume personal responsibility for one's self, communicate with colleagues, break down complex tasks into steps, and work through those steps successfully. Halpern noted that when youth focus with peers in this way, they learn to transcend their differences of race, culture, age, and clique, as well as the sense of insecurity that is common at this age. Furthermore, they are able to see themselves in a larger context, beyond their social group, school, or community.

Positive relationships

"Perhaps the most robust research finding in human development is that experiencing support from the people in one's environment, from infancy on, has broad impacts on later functioning."[3] The TASC study found that the program promoted the formation of strong, positive relationships between the participants, and between participants and the adult staff, many of whom were teachers. As a result of these experiences, participants saw their teachers in a different light, reexamined the positive role that school could play in their future success, and expanded their vision of what they themselves were capable of accomplishing. Speaking about the teachers who stay after the end of the school day to work in the after-school program, one student at a TASC program said, "As a result of being in the program, you appreciate [the teachers] more. . . . After I saw the way [Mr. S.] was with us, I started respecting him as a person . . . and as a teacher. Now I go to class more. . . . He's my best teacher."

Successful implementation: Lessons learned

Older youth place much higher demands on program providers than younger youth, which makes attracting them and retaining their participation challenging. This is especially true for those just starting up or attempting to replicate models developed for younger children. Although not all of the programs in the initiatives are showing the same success, they have generated valuable lessons to those interested in expanding their programming to older youth.

Building relationships

Our collective experiences highlight the truism that youth "may come for the activity but they stay for the relationships."[4] But why are some programs successful and others not? Obviously, hiring the right staff is key: staff members who enjoy working with older youth in a relaxed, informal setting, can quickly establish trust, and authentically mix encouragement and praise with honest feedback and guidance. To make good hiring decisions, some programs ask applicants to lead an activity with actual program participants, who later rate their performance and participate in the final hiring decisions. No one has an automatic pass, even classroom teachers who enjoy the privileges of seniority during the school day.

Hiring the right staff, however, is not always enough. Ensuring the building of positive relationships requires that young people have access to these adults. Many successful programs ensure that staff members are accessible by providing unstructured time to interact with youth, free from the responsibilities of leading formal activities. Sometimes this means accepting a challenge game of checkers or taking a walk across the campus with a young person.

Because access to adults also means that youth know where to find them, making dedicated space is one of the most important variables for program success. With dedicated space, staff and participants can create an identity and youth space on campus that declares that "something new is happening here." It can serve as a drop-in center throughout the day; could be furnished with computers, books, board games, lockers, and even refrigerators and microwave ovens; and can be used by students during study hall, lunch, or while waiting for activities to begin. Often this space embodies a commitment to youth and adult partnership, as the staff and youth leaders work side by side, without the barriers of walls or partitions. To build a sense of community within a large, sprawling campus, some projects schedule as many activities as they can in classrooms adjacent to the after-school office, establishing a solid hub for the program.

Relevance and mastery

More so than younger teens, high school youth are looking for programs relevant to their interests and related to the real world that awaits them. "The idea of 'high school afterschool programming' is an oxymoron if one's image of afterschool activities involves 11-year-olds munching snacks, getting help with their homework and finding creative outlets for their energy until their parents arrive at 6 P.M."[5]

Relevance. The best way to identify what will be interesting and relevant to older youth is to gather their thoughts and involve them in programming decisions. When asked, youth always voice the need to make money and support themselves outside school. As a result, many programs focus on helping youth begin building bridges to the world of work by promoting the development of soft skills through hands-on, project-based activities. Soft skills include the ability to communicate with coworkers, work as a team member, meet expectations, problem-solve, and work in multicultural settings. In ASM programs, students are expected to produce real-world products after only ten weeks of working together. These products may include public murals, Web sites designed for nonprofit organizations, or digital videos promoting positive messages. In an observational study of one ASM program, Reed Larson found that teens "came to recognize that exchanges between self and others facilitated their work" and that "what seemed to be emergent for these youth was a grasp of the complementarity between self and others as members of a collaborative system working toward an instrumental goal."[6]

After-school programs can also provide youth with opportunities to develop technical skills in areas such as videography, graphic arts, Web design, robotics, and those related to the visual and performing arts. Finally, many programs offer work-based learning opportunities such as job shadowing and work internships, which often lead to paid employment during the school year and summer.

Moving from engagement to mastery. In her study of the San Francisco Beacon Centers, Milbrey McLaughlin found that "across sites, students valued activities that gave them the opportunities to develop skills that mattered to them. . . . Furthermore, it wasn't just the opportunity to dabble in these activities: youth talked about the importance of opportunities where they actually learned something or improved in a domain of interest."[7] It is through these experiences that participants are able to see their progress as they attempt, practice, attain, and master new skills. "Recognition of one's capacity to work hard, combined with growth in specific skills, feedback on specific work, and the creation of real products, contribute to a more genuine self-regard."[8] As one ASM teen said, "Something that's fun, it will help get your self-esteem up 'cause you'll be doing all this cool stuff that you never thought you'd be able to do, like putting on a dance or a play and you can look back and be like I did that."

Instructors

Being "cool" and able to relate to older youth is not enough. Older youth respect adults who are masters at what they do, and these are the people they want to learn from. Thus, successful programs often enlist instructors who are highly qualified professionals in their field and know how to empower others with their knowledge. In the words of one youth, "Competence is more important than cool!" If running a digital video program, a cinematographer or someone with a similar background should be hired over a classroom teacher who can operate a video camera. If young people do not believe that their instructor has the expertise to teach them the skills necessary for success in the real world, it will be difficult to ensure their ongoing participation.

Serious outcomes requires serious partnerships

After-school programs that are located on school campuses are uniquely positioned to have a significant impact on young people's academic success. For youth who are more seriously disengaged, after-school programs can help them connect their interest to subjects outside school. For some youth, this becomes a compelling reason to attend and do better in school. Making this happen is not easy and certainly cannot be done without the serious attention and partnership of school decision makers and teachers.

School leadership

Partnership with the school leadership is critical if the after-school program is to contribute to the broader school mission. This means more than passive permission to share space on the campus. Programs need to be considered a full stakeholder and contributor to the school's success or failure. "School is here from 8:00 AM to 6:00 PM. What does that mean? It means enrichment, remediation and college activities are attached to or in collaboration with our after school program," said a TASC principal.

In the more successful after-school programs, the program leader is a member of the senior management team, attends all of the teaching staff meetings, and has a standing item on the agenda. In these schools, the principal is a strong champion of the program, conferences with the program director on a regular basis, and knocks down institutional barriers when they are marginalizing the effects of the program. Establishing full integration with a school takes time. Having a presence on campus during the regular school day, with the ability to attend key meetings during and after school, requires the commitment of a full-time director.

Identifying young people in need

Strong integration with the school means that program leaders have access to teachers and data to identify young people who are not on track to graduate due to failing classes, the lack of necessary credits, or past failure on district exams. By having specific and updated information on each student, after-school leaders are able to work in partnership with youth to establish clear academic goals and track progress on a regular basis.

Focus on graduation

Ensuring that young people are on track toward graduation requires more than homework help and study hall. Programs that are making a difference are offering a range of academic supports, including content-based tutoring in needed academic areas, especially math and science, and opportunities to make up labs missed during the school day. Many are also offering test preparation for major exams, state high school exit exams, benchmark tests, and SAT preparation.

Even if program participants are currently passing the required tests, they will not graduate if they have lost credits in earlier years. One program employs retired high school teachers to conduct classes after school, allowing youth to retrieve lost credits. Other programs are authorized by the school to offer high school elective credits for consistent participation in standards-based after-school projects. In one California high school, 63 percent of the 2005 graduates earned some of their needed school credits in the after-school program, boosting the school's graduation rate to the highest in twenty years.[9]

Recommendations for policymakers and funders

The after-school movement has largely ignored older youth. Although they represent a sizable percentage of American students, they garner only a small fraction of the federal state and local investments for after-school programs. This is partly due to beliefs that older youth will not stay at school to participate in these programs, especially those who are identified as most in need. With the documented success of programs within the initiatives surveyed here and some early evaluation findings, these myths are now being dispelled. Emerging from these pioneering efforts are some promising practices and program models that can guide the development of future afterschool programs but not without the help of policymakers and funders, both public and private. Some recommendations for policymakers and funders follow.

Level of funding

Properly designed and implemented high school after-school programs can attract and support improved outcomes for older youth. However, there is little funding available. Policymakers should seek to increase available multiyear funding of these programs and plan on increasing funding as we consolidate our learnings about what works and as program models show positive impact.

Program accountability

After-school programming for high school youth is relatively new, and it is important that funders not ask programs to overpromise as to their process or participant outcomes or the time frames needed to achieve these outcomes. Early outcomes should be realistic, with ample time to align the program with the culture of the school. If expectations of improved academic outcomes are included, they should be tangible and measurable and shared by the youth participants. A good example is improved graduation rates; a poor example is raising standardized test scores. In addition, funders and policymakers should begin to rely less on traditional measures and instead help after-school programs measure the things they are actually affecting, such as hard and soft skills.

Promoting program quality

Resources to support program improvement must be provided. These resources should include convening program leaders to learn from one another, case studies of successful programs that highlight creative practices and strategies, formative and outcome evaluations, and access to technical assistance and training opportunities.

Ensuring access to diverse opportunities

Older youth need access to diverse learning opportunities if they are to make a successful transition to adulthood. These opportunities come from programs that provide a range of intensive skill-building experiences over a fixed period of time, as well as those that offer ongoing, comprehensive support. Some are best located on school sites, while others ensure access by being located in neighborhood youth agencies. Because we know that one size does not fit all, it is important that policymakers and funders support a diversity of learning opportunities for older youth.

Notes

1. California Department of Education. (2006). *Funding results: 21st Century Community Learning Center: High Schools.* Retrieved January 24, 2006, from http://www.cde.ca.gov/fg/fo/r8/cclchs05result.asp.

2. Halpern, R. (in press). After school matters in Chicago: Apprenticeship as a model for youth programming. *Journal of Youth and Society.*

3. Gambone, M. A., Klem, A. M., & Connell, J. P. (2002). *Finding out what matters for youth development.* Philadelphia: Youth Development Strategies and Institute for Research and Reform in Education. Retrieved January 24, 2006, from www.ydsi.org/YDSI/pdf/WhatMatters.pdf.

4. Yohalem, N., Wilson-Ahlstrom, A., & Pittman, K. (2005, August). *Out of school time policy commentary #10: Rethinking the high school experience: What's after school got to do with it?* Washington, DC: Forum for Youth Investment, Impact Strategies. Retrieved January 1, 2006, from http://www.forumfyi.org/Files/ostpc10.pdf.

5. Forum for Youth Investment. (2004, February). *High school: The next frontier for after-school advocates?* Washington, DC: Forum for Youth Investment, Impact Strategies. Retrieved January 1, 2006, from http://www.forumfyi.org/Files//ForumFOCUS_Feb2004.pdf.

6. Larson, R. (in press). From "I" to "We": Development of the capacity for teamwork in youth programs. In R. Silbereisen & R. Lerner (Eds.), *Approaches to positive youth development.* Thousand Oaks, CA: Sage.

7. McLaughlin, M. (2003). Youth voices on learning after school. In *A Qualitative Evaluation of the San Francisco Beacon Initiative: Executive Summary* (pp. 1–8). Palo Alto, CA: Stanford University School of Education. Retrieved January 20, 2006, from http://www.cnyd.org/home/YouthVoicesReport.pdf#search=%22YOUTH%20VOICES%2C%20BEACONS%22.

8. Halpern. (in press).

9. Fennessy, B., & Bocia, R. (2005, September). *Blair High School and Pasadena LEARNs program: Students are walking the walk.* Pasadena LEARNs press release, Pasadena, CA.

SARAH BARR *is an evaluation specialist for After School Matters in Chicago.*

JENNIFER BIRMINGHAM *is a senior research associate at Policy Studies Associates in Washington, D.C.*

JENNIFER FORNAL *is the former project manager at the Community Network for Youth Development and is currently working as an independent consultant in San Francisco.*

RACHEL KLEIN *is the senior director of research and evaluation at After School Matters in Chicago.*

SAM PIHA *is the former director for the Community School Partnerships at the Community Network for Youth Development in San Francisco and is currently an independent consultant in the areas of high school reform and youth development.*

Social action theory provides a valuable youth engagement strategy that emphasizes youth voice, participatory practice, and community building.

6

Young people and social action: Youth participation in the United Kingdom and United States

Joan Arches, Jennie Fleming

TOWARD THE END of the twentieth century, the idea that young people are social actors gained increasing predominance. Since then, there has been a growing recognition of young people's ability to understand and contribute to forming their environments.

One demonstration of this is the ratification of the United Nations Convention on the Rights of the Child (UNCRC) by most of the countries of the world (though not the United States). The UNCRC made children's rights part of the social contract. Article 12 of the UNCRC specifically addresses the rights of children, as citizens, to be represented and participate in decisions affecting their lives.

In this chapter, we discuss the state of youth participation in the United Kingdom and United States and then describe two

This chapter could not have been written without the work and enthusiasm of the young people involved in the social action groups in England and America. We thank them and wish them well.

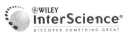

projects—one in each country—that represent efforts to stimulate young people's initiative in working for community change. The principles of social action, as developed by the Centre for Social Action, informed both of these projects. The projects demonstrate how social action practice can be a valuable framework for youth engagement. It emphasizes youth voice, participatory practice, and community building. Older youth consistently point to these components as necessary and desirable features of youth organizations and projects. Project examples help us to understand the challenges and tasks of using the social action framework to inspire youth leadership and healthy development.

Young people and participation

The emergence of the idea that young people should be involved in decisions that affect their lives has been becoming more central in both public debate and government policies in the United Kingdom. Prout suggests that "in part its emergence has to do with a more general shift in institutional practice that affected children and adults alike. Rapid social change has eroded and fragmented once taken-for-granted institutions and has led to a new sense of uncertainty and risk."[1] This has led to a need for organizations and institutions to be more responsive and flexible, seeking the views and opinions of those affected by their policies.

A commitment to young people's participation is increasingly embedded in government policy and practice in the United Kingdom. The Department for Education and Skills (DfES) produced a document called *Listening to Learn*, which states, "Our vision is for a department which is young–person friendly and accessible, responsive to their needs and aspirations, and renowned throughout government for leading change in involving children and young people."[2] An earlier government document "sets out the expectation that ten national Governmental departments would develop action plans promoting the participation of children and young people in their core mission and work."[3] This is the context for youth participation in the United Kingdom today.

But while the current emphasis on young people's participation in Britain is on young people being encouraged by adults to join in with formal structures often based on notions of representative democracy, concepts of young people as citizens and involvement in governance are developing, but these still tend to be framed by adults. The more participative form of democracy, based on young people campaigning for community change as in social action, is frequently lacking. Thus, this chapter contributes to the reinvigoration of this practice and seeks to act as a stimulus for its further development.

Although the United States was one of the two countries that did not sign the UNCRC, for many Americans in the field of youth work, there is a commitment to participatory practice for which social action may be of considerable relevance.

The past twenty years have seen a steady stream of work based on youth assets, youth as community builders, and youth leadership that emphasizes strengths, participation, and the importance of youth having their voices heard. As part of the positive youth development approach, among others, youth inclusion is seen as key to policy, programs, planning, and practice with young people. There are now more youth than in the past who are involved in community-based initiatives and have the potential to change their lives and improve their communities.

Educators, researchers, and practitioners using practice perspectives based on participatory methodologies such as participatory action research, asset-based organizing, and participatory planning have moved the field forward. For educators and practitioners in the United States committed to youth participation, social action provides a theory and practice that enhances community building, social cohesion, and positive youth development.

Nevertheless, there is still much to learn about working with youth to facilitate their taking charge of their situations and taking responsibility for their behavior. Social action holds promise in these areas.

NEW DIRECTIONS FOR YOUTH DEVELOPMENT • DOI: 10.1002/yd

Social action

As practiced by the Centre for Social Action (CSA), social action is a specific philosophy and theory for social change based on the work of Paolo Freire,[4] influenced by the disability movement,[5] black activists,[6] and the women's movement.[7] Social action emerged in the late 1970s as a distinctive value-based group practice, with a focus on social justice, rights, and empowerment. It focuses on working with groups and changing unequal power relations, while creating opportunities for improving conditions in their environment.

As a value-based practice, the CSA has six explicitly stated principles that guide its work. The first of the principles affirms a commitment to work for social justice. The second asserts that all people have skills, knowledge, and experience that they can use to address problems they face. Third, people have the right to be heard, define the issues that are facing them, and take action on their own behalf. The fourth principle recognizes that oppression and injustice are complex issues rooted in social and economic practices and policy. Fifth, social action is concerned with facilitating a process whereby people collectively learn to discover those parts of their lives that they can change. There is a recognition that social change can most effectively be carried out within the context of a group and that individuals are more powerful when they act collectively. Social action is group action. The sixth principle states that professionals are not to act as experts but as facilitators in a social change process. (For more information, see www.dmu.ac.uk/dmucsa.)

In addition to its values base, social action fuses process and outcome; both are equally important. Social action is about attempting to create learning and change; it is not seeking solely individual outcomes. While participants determine and control the content of their agenda and actions, the social action methodology guides the process.

CSA staff members (usually two workers who facilitate the group and then meet with an outside consultant between group sessions) work with groups to facilitate a five-part process in which participants (1) identify problems or issues, (2) analyze why these conditions or issues exist, (3) figure out how to address them, (4) carry out an action, and (5) engage in reflection. Asking "why" is essential in social action, as it creates a vehicle to collectively analyze the root causes of the problems. The workers encourage reflection and pose questions as integral parts of all meetings.

For youth to become effective, active citizens, they require opportunities to learn and use skills in decision making, participation, and civic engagement. Social action encourages young people to use these opportunities with a view toward creating change at a number of levels. While change in the community in which the young people live is the most important change from a social action point of view, it may also happen at an individual, group, or societal level. The two case studies that follow illuminate this approach.

Braunstone: Young People's Research and Development Project

The example from the United Kingdom took place in a low-income community in a Midlands city. The youth were predominantly white, aged eight to fifteen, and living in the same community. As part of New Deal for Communities, the CSA was employed to work with young people to find out what they thought about their living conditions and what they thought New Deal money should be spent on. New Deal for Communities (NDC) is a "key programme in the Government's strategy to tackle multiple deprivation in the most deprived neighbourhoods in the country, giving some of the poorest communities the resources to tackle their problems in an intensive and co-ordinated way."[8]

For this project, it was important to work in a way that encouraged the youth to take part and share what they knew with others in New Deal Braunstone. Staff recruited, trained, and supported six project workers aged eighteen to twenty-five from the community. Every effort was made to include views of young people, especially those who might not normally get the chance to have their voices heard. The project workers spent time going to places where they knew young people would be—in the street, the parks, and outside shops. The project started by bringing fifty young people to De Montfort University. The young people worked in groups, gave themselves a name, and started to work on explaining what it was like to be a young person living in Braunstone.

After the first meeting, the young people divided into four groups, and the local project workers met with each group once a week. They considered what was good and bad about Braunstone. They created drawings and posters, took photos, and made lists. They considered why the issues existed and why they needed changing. From a large list of issues that they felt affected their lives (and the lives of others; many of the issues were not exclusive to young people), the young people had to negotiate priorities to present to New Deal. Their lists included cleaning up the area, removing burned-out houses and cars, cleaning out a pond in the park, stopping syringes being left in parks, lighting, taking action on crime, robberies and guns, and clubs and activities for young people.

The groups also consulted with a wider group of young people to find out what they thought of their priorities and suggestions for change. They presented their findings in song, photos, and posters.

When these youth spoke about the impact of their participation in the project, they indicated that they felt empowered by their new ability to speak and be heard. Increased self-pride, the importance of the group, and the feelings that they could make a difference and could get results emerged from their comments:

When people bring stuff to New Deal, like say we wanted a swing built on the park, we'd know what to say to them. We know how to ask.

At school when you get people coming in, like the council and the police, you know what to say to them. It gives you confidence to talk to them.

Seeing the group as a positive alternative to their school experiences and acceptance by workers were themes echoed by these youth—for example: "It is more fun than school, it gives an opportunity to do things differently."

They felt they had learned to use new skills, had greater self-confidence, and had a more focused outlook as a result of participating in the social action process. All the youth referred to the communication and group skills they developed as a result of this project. "We've learnt how to compromise; to work in groups and respect each other," said one.

The group felt they had made an impact on their community in terms of making the community safer and cleaner. One person reflected, "I think we've improved other people's lives. . . . That's why we came into the group. That's why we don't want it to end. We've worked hard and we want to sort Braunstone out."

The comments indicated that the social action work had resulted in some change at the personal, group, and community levels. Two key points the young people made about the social action group were choice and inclusion. They recognized that in their social action group, everybody could become involved and participate. It was important for the group that they were able to choose the activities and set the agenda and that even when the group facilitators asked the group to engage in something, there was always room for discussion.

Healthy Initiative Collaborative: Community University Partnership

This case from the United States is based on a three-year service-learning collaborative project between the College of Public and Community Service at the University of Massachusetts, Boston; the Geiger Gibson Community Health Center; and Walter Denney Youth Center. Healthy Initiative Collaborative: Community University Partnership (HIC CUP) includes a diverse group of low-income youth ages nine to seventeen, who reside at Harbor Point, a private for-profit, mixed-income housing development located next to the university on a relatively isolated peninsula. Similar to Braunstone, the purpose of the project has been for the youth to become community researchers and problem solvers. By working in partnership with the university students, the objective has been to engage the youth in a highly meaningful civic engagement project.

NEW DIRECTIONS FOR YOUTH DEVELOPMENT • DOI: 10.1002/yd

HIC CUP youth began thinking about their community by participating in an exercise in which they envisioned themselves as filmmakers who had just completed a documentary on their community. They were asked to draw the poster advertising the film. For many, this was the first time they thought about their community in a systematic way. They shared their posters, telling each other why they had included specific items. This led to discussion followed by more research as the youth went out with cameras to take pictures of their community. Coming back once again, they shared their findings and made new posters. During this time, they developed project ownership by naming themselves the Harbor Point Community Research Unit (HPCRU).

Once they identified concerns, they went on to find out if other youth in the neighborhood agreed. The youth, in partnership with the university students, learned about and designed surveys to administer to other youth. Their analysis of the data from a hundred surveys revealed that trash, lack of recreational opportunities, and harassment by security were the three major concerns. These were the same as those earlier identified by HPCRU. Using force-field analysis, HPCRU made the decision to select the need for recreational activities as their project. Having identified the *what*, they spent several weeks discussing *why* there were so few recreational outlets for them. Their discussions included talk about how they felt stereotyped based in part on the way they dressed. They felt the stereotypes portrayed them as bad. They also felt racism played a part in the stereotypes and in the resulting treatment they had experienced. The youth felt they were ignored and their needs dismissed.

This fruitful discussion of *why* enabled them to move on to the next step in which they spent their time figuring out how they would address the problem—the *how* stage of the social action process. After deciding to work for a basketball court, they developed a proposal, created a logo, collected four hundred signatures on petitions, raised funds, generated publicity, and presented their proposal to others for support.

Throughout this process, they have been learning to make their voices heard. They have held community meetings, met with leadership, and are now known at Harbor Point. They have learned where power resides in their community and how to address those in power. At the end of one semester, the youth were asked what they learned so far from the project. The following quotes reflect their answers:

The group motivates us to help our community and to keep us off the streets.

The group has kept me out of trouble.

When the young people were asked, "What was something positive you learned about yourself through your work here?" they gave a variety of answers that included:

HIC CUP is about community in need of help from young kids and that we can make a difference.

I learned how to create a group and work together to help the community.

It gets you thinking, gives you skills (kids can make a difference).

Conclusion

Neither of these case studies depicts an unbridled success. The U.S. example is ongoing, and we do not yet know if they will be successful in getting the basketball court. And the U.K. example did not result in the continued involvement of youth. Once the CSA was no longer involved after the young people had presented their findings and report, the New Deal did not continue with the participation of young people.

Nevertheless, both case studies show how committed young people can be in working to improve their neighborhoods. They show that social action as a youth engagement strategy can enable young people to identify the issues that are important to them, determine why they exist, and consider a plan for change. From our experiences, we believe that social action has much to offer to those committed to working with youth to promote the participation and leadership of young people in the communities in which they live.[9]

Notes

1. Prout, A. (2003). Participation, policy and the changing conditions of childhood. In C. Hallett & A. Prout (Eds.), *Hearing the voices of children: Social policy for a new century.* London: Routledge Falmer.
2. Department for Education and Skills. (2002). *Listening to learn (summary).* Sheffield: Department for Education and Skills.
3. Badham, B. (2004). Participation—for a change: Disabled young people lead the way. *Children and Society, 18*(2), 143–155.
4. Freire, P. (1970). *Pedagogy of the oppressed.* New York: Seabury Press.
5. Oliver, M. (1992). Changing the social relations of research production. *Disability, Handicap and Society, 7*(2), 101–114.
6. Gilroy, P. (1987). *There ain't no black in the Union Jack.* London: Hutchinson; hooks, b. (1992). *Ain't I a woman: Black women and feminism.* London: Pluto Press.
7. Dominelli, L., & McCleod, E. (1989). *Feminist social work.* London: Macmillan; Evans, M. (Ed.). (1994). *The woman question.* Thousand Oaks, CA: Sage.
8. Neighborhood Renewal Unit. (n.d.). *New Deal for Communities.* Retrieved January 7, 2005, from http://www.neighbourhood.gov.uk/page.asp?id=617.
9. For those interested in finding out more about how to facilitate young people in undertaking social action projects, the following resource might be helpful: National Writing Project. (2006). *Writing for a change.* San Francisco: Jossey-Bass.

JOAN ARCHES *is associate professor at the College of Public and Community Service, University of Massachusetts, Boston.*

JENNIE FLEMING *is the director of the Centre for Social Action, De Montfort University, Leicester, United Kingdom.*

*Recent research and evaluation of youth develop-
ment and employment programs suggests that the
demands of the knowledge economy and the emerging digital economy are causing employers to expect
higher levels of skills from older youth.*

7

Workforce development for older youth

David E. Brown, Mala B. Thakur

THE CHALLENGES FACING YOUTH who are disconnected from our
nation's employment and education systems are expansive. Studies
by the Center for Labor Market Studies at Northeastern University indicate that employment prospects for youth between the ages
of sixteen and nineteen have decreased in the past three years
despite overall job growth. The 2004 youth employment rate of
36.4 percent was lowest in the fifty-seven years these data have been
collected. From 2000 to 2004, the employment-to-population ratio
of employed teens declined by 8.8 percentage points.[1]

On the education front, research that the Urban Institute conducted in 2004 on graduation rates revealed that the national public high school graduation rate is only 68 percent, with nearly a

Parts of this chapter have been borrowed with permission from 39 *Clearinghouse Review*
229 (July-Aug. 2005). © 2005 Sargent Shriver National Center on Poverty Law. The
views expressed in this chapter are solely those of the authors.

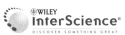

third of all public high school students failing to graduate. This report also underscored the racial gaps in graduation rates, with students from minority groups (American Indian, Hispanic, and African American) having little more than a fifty-fifty chance of earning a high school diploma.[2] Similarly, juvenile offenders and youth who are aging out of foster care have very low high school completion rates and face significant challenges to gainful and legal employment.

In today's labor market, opportunities for employment at a living wage, and ultimately self-sufficiency, are dismal for those who lack the higher level of skills demanded by employers. The twenty-first-century labor market is unforgiving. In the years ahead, over 75 percent of new jobs will require postsecondary education or training.[3] Many employers are increasingly relying on immigrant labor, outsourcing, and outplacement overseas to meet their labor needs.[4]

This chapter provides some insights into strategies that have been implemented to facilitate older youth's transitions to the workforce and highlights the supports youth need for successful adulthood, citizenship, and career pursuits.

History of federal investments in youth workforce development

The federal Comprehensive Employment and Training Act (CETA) was amended in 1978 to include the massive and ambitious Youth Employment Demonstration Projects Act.[5] Many of these programs were a response to social and economic issues that were highlighted throughout the previous decade. In 1982, the Job Training Partnership Act (JTPA) replaced CETA. Under JTPA, funding was cut significantly, and employment and training programs were more narrowly focused on job placement and meeting the needs of employers. Many programs targeting youth were eliminated. Lower costs and high placement rates were mandated; hence, youth work experience (except for the Summer Youth Employment Program) and long-term services to youth were reduced significantly. The enactment of JTPA was based on the assumption that "state and local decision-making were better than federal decision-making and that business knew best what priorities and programs would be most effective."[6]

Research conducted in the 1990s suggested that youth services and supports that are grounded in a developmental approach not only helped young people avoid self-destructive behavior, but also enabled them to acquire the academic and work-readiness skills and personal attributes employers sought. The research profiled in *Some Things Do Make a Difference* included studies of Big Brother Big Sisters, the Quantum Opportunities Program, the Center for Employment Training, the Service and Conservation Corps, and Job Corps.[7] Taken together, the research recommended the implementation of comprehensive and long-term youth development initiatives.

The Workforce Investment Act of 1998 (WIA), which repealed JTPA, reflects much of what had been learned from the recent research about how to prepare young people for adulthood.[8] WIA mandates the creation of coordinated, effective, and customer-focused workforce development and employment services. The youth provisions of WIA require states and localities to provide a comprehensive workforce preparation system that reflects the developmental needs of youth. Implementation of the WIA therefore provided an opportunity for states and communities to begin to combine traditional youth employment and training services with activities grounded in the principles of youth development. WIA acknowledges the consensus that emerged from both research and practice that preparing youth for careers and adult roles requires more than the narrow range of training-related services that had commonly been provided by youth employment and training programs.[9] WIA also directs states to make intentional efforts to engage youth within the juvenile justice and foster care systems. Congress is once again looking to reauthorize WIA. It is expected that the reauthorized WIA youth program will be targeted more toward out-of-school and more vulnerable youth, including juvenile offenders, foster youth, and youth with disabilities. It also may incorporate new program elements, including financial literacy and on the job training.

─────────────

What works? The Promising and Effective Practices Network

In 1995, the National Youth Employment Coalition (NYEC) and its members established the Promising and Effective Practices Network (PEPNet) to identify the key elements of quality youth programs and develop tools that would help organizations establish, connect to, and promote quality programs.[10] PEPNet represents a standards framework that captures the key elements common to successful programs that connect youth to jobs, careers, and education. Building on this framework, NYEC developed a range of information and tools, and PEPNet became the major resource in the United States on what works in programs that connect young people ages fourteen to twenty-five to work, careers, and education.

In the past ten years, thousands of youth professionals around the United States and internationally have used PEPNet.[11] PEPNet has informed a movement to increase quality of youth programming; has raised the visibility of successful youth employment programs; and has influenced policies, including the Workforce Investment Act, to reflect what has been learned that works for youth. By promoting high standards and quality practices, PEPNet raised the bar on performance and enabled youth-related organizations to maximize their resources by focusing on what has been proven to work. NYEC augmented the framework with new research and with practices of ninety-six PEPNet-awarded programs, selected in an annual, national, peer-reviewed recognition process.

PEPNet has identified four key areas that are common to successful programs: (1) strong management, (2) a comprehensive programmatic approach to working with youth, (3) a focus on building competencies that will help youth succeed in education and work, and (4) measurement of the success they have with youth.

NEW DIRECTIONS FOR YOUTH DEVELOPMENT • DOI: 10.1002/yd

Management for quality

When looking for a quality program, the first thing to assess is its management. Without strong management practices and systems, a program lacks the foundation to provide effective services for youth.

Programmatic approach

The organizations that are most successful in connecting youth with work and education design their programs with structures in place to support a comprehensive approach:

- Environment and culture: Does the program have a safe, structured environment that supports young people's development and transition to adulthood?
- Instructional approach: Throughout its activities, does the program employ active, hands-on instructional strategies? Do youth have opportunities to reflect on their learning?
- Targeting youth: Can the program easily tell who it serves? Is the length of program activities and the intensity (that is, number of hours a week) appropriate for youth to accomplish work- and education-related goals?
- Collaboration: Does the program partner with other organizations to expand the services it can offer youth?
- Individual planning: Is a plan for the program experience developed with each young person based on his or her strengths and needs and revisited regularly?
- Wraparound support: Does the program provide or connect youth to needed personal supports beyond education and training? Does it engage family members or other positive adults in the youth's life?
- Youth engagement: Does the program engage youth as active, respected contributors?
- Employer engagement: To ensure program activities are relevant to actual workplace needs, does the program actively engage public and private sector employers?
- Transition support: Does the program gradually move youth from full program participation to independent engagement in

positive activities such as work or education? Does it have transition activities and supports for at least a year? Does it work with alumni?

Youth development competencies

Programs are most successful if they do not focus on just one area, such as work. Rather, they help youth build the range of competencies: skills, knowledge, or abilities that will help them successfully make the transition to work and adulthood.

From a range of youth development research, NYEC found that youth need to develop competencies in five areas:

• Working: Does the program help youth develop competencies to find employment, such as résumé writing, interviewing, and job searching? Do youth develop competencies to maintain employment, such as communication, interpersonal, and decision-making skills? Do youth experience work or worklike environments through internships, community service, job shadows, or other opportunities?

• Academic learning: Does the program help young people increase their literacy and numeracy skills? Does it help them progress toward a recognized credential like a high school diploma or general equivalency diploma (GED)? Are the youth connected to pathways to postsecondary education or training?

• Connecting: Does the program develop relationships between youth participants and caring adults? Does it foster positive peer group relationships? Does it promote acceptance of diverse groups and help youth learn how to work cooperatively?

• Leading: Does the program provide structured opportunities for all participants to lead, such as contributing to program oversight, contributing to the community, leading participant teams or activities, or in other ways?

• Thriving: Does the program promote healthy decision making and take steps to divert youth engagement in risky behaviors? Does it help youth access health-related services and develop independent living skills?

Quality programs intentionally help youth build competencies in each of these areas, but specific activities depend on the program's purpose and youth served. Most programs cannot provide activities in all competency areas, but they can develop partnership and referral relationships with complementary organizations. Research shows that increases in competencies are associated with increased well-being.

Evidence of success

A critical element of quality programs is that they achieve positive results with youth. The PEPNet outcomes are aligned with common measures used by the federal government, demonstrating skills attainment, academic achievement, credential attainment, and productive engagement and retention over time in employment and postsecondary education and training.[12] However, it is important to recognize that these outcomes do not demonstrate all that participants achieve in youth programs. Because so much of the effort in youth programs is spent in activities that lead up to these final outcomes or are related to harder-to-measure youth development competencies, it is important to identify and measure a series of progress measures that show relative gains over time. The inclusion of progress measures both encourages and enables programs to document and demonstrate the incremental gains young people make as a result of participation in the program, such as passing a GED section test, completing a community service project, establishing positive peer relationships, or serving in a leadership position.

Opportunities, supports, and services in preparation for work

Recent research and evaluation of youth development and employment programs suggest that the demands of the knowledge economy and the emerging digital economy are causing employers to expect higher levels of skills from youth. These changes require that programs expand the mix of services they provide by:

- Increasing academic rigor and improving academic performance
- Teaching SCANS (Secretary's Commission on Achieving Necessary Skills) skills such as interpersonal, thinking, resource, and information-gathering skills
- Shifting from process-focused evaluations to outcome accountability
- Expanding the use of effective holistic approaches, such as the integration of academics, vocational education, and work-based learning and the use of an array of technologies
- Involving employers more intensively in the education system
- Obtaining and applying better information on the skill requirements of particular occupations
- Strengthening the transition from high school to postsecondary education, especially for students who have not traditionally continued their education after high school[13]

Through a literature review of promising practices focused on the needs of youth ages fourteen to twenty-five, NYEC and the national collaboration have identified a range of opportunities, supports, and services that all youth need in order to meet the higher level of skills discussed above, including additional opportunities, supports, and services for youth with disabilities. A set of common operating principles was developed based on what all youth need in the transition from adolescence to productive adulthood and citizenship, including making informed choices about what career paths they want to pursue. Youth need all of the following:

High-quality standards-based education regardless of setting
- Academic programs based on clear state standards
- Career and technical education programs based on professional and industry standards

- Curricular and program options based on universal design of school, work, and community-based learning experiences
- Learning environments that are small and safe
- Supports from highly qualified staff
- Access to an assessment system that includes multiple measures
- Graduation standards that include options

Preparatory experiences

- Career assessment, including interest inventories and formal and informal vocational assessments
- Information about career opportunities that provide a living wage, including information about education, entry requirements, and income potential
- Training in job-seeking skills
- Structured exposure to postsecondary education and other life-long learning opportunities

Work-based experiences

- Opportunities to engage in a range of work-based exploration activities such as site visits and job shadowing
- Multiple on-the-job training experiences, including community service (paid or unpaid) that is specifically linked to the content of a program of study

Youth development and youth leadership opportunities

- Mentoring activities designed to establish strong relationships with adults through formal and informal settings
- Exposure to role models in a variety of contexts
- Training in skills such as self-advocacy and conflict resolution
- Exposure to personal leadership and youth development activities, including community service
- Opportunities to exercise leadership

Connecting activities to support services

- Mental and physical health services
- Transportation

- Tutoring
- Postprogram supports through structured arrangements in post-secondary institutions and adult service agencies
- Connections to other services and opportunities such as recreation[14]

Looking forward

The work described in this chapter suggests the progress made to support youth school-to-work transitions through the stalwart commitment and decades of hard work of many individuals, organizations, and benefactors. It reflects the growth of a diverse coalition of nearly three hundred organizations that under the aegis of NYEC seek to educate policymakers and to support service providers on behalf of our nation's youth. Fortunately, like the young people we all serve, the work of the coalition and other youth-serving organizations will continue to evolve to meet the challenges and address the conditions that undermine the aspirations of far too many youth.

Additional resources

This section includes more detailed information on PEPNet resources, including Quality Standards, the Online Index, and several related measurement tools.

Guides

The *PEPNet Guide to Quality Standards for Youth Programs: Linking Youth to Work and Education for a Successful Transition to Adulthood* details the PEPNet Standards and serves as the basic reference source for the updated PEPNet. It answers frequently asked questions about PEPNet and explains how to tap into PEPNet's resources to improve the quality of youth programming. It also provides examples of how the standards work in practice, drawn from programs that PEPNet has recognized for quality.

The guide is intended to build the ability of youth programs to measure and document performance. In an easy-to-use, easy-to-understand format, the book covers the basics of selecting and measuring outcomes; types of data that programs should track based on PEPNet's outcomes and progress measures; methods for collecting and managing data; and how to use data for continuous improvement. It also provides guidance for funders and policymakers on understanding, selecting, and documenting results.

Online Index

The upgraded Online Index to Quality Practices includes over a thousand specific quality practices identified from nationally recognized, PEPNet-awarded youth programs. The index makes it possible for users to search for information by a specific PEPNet quality standard or indicator, practice (examples include follow-up, staff development, youth leadership, and employer engagement), youth population served (including urban or rural), program funding stream, organization, or any key word the user chooses. The index is linked to PEPNet Awardee Profiles, in-depth descriptions of the structure and practices of programs that received the PEPNet Award for quality practices between 1999 and 2003.

Tools

The PEPNet Quality Self Assessment Tool enables multiple program staff and other stakeholders to complete the PEPNet Quality Self Assessment electronically. Each individual rates an organization on how well it currently satisfies each of the PEPNet Standards and respective indicators. The new online capability provides numerous benefits. For example, individuals may complete the assessment at their own pace, saving responses and going back to edit or finish another time. The system automatically provides a report of the cumulative responses, making it easy to debrief and identify areas for improvement. The site provides all the information needed to complete the assessment, including step-by-step instructions on administering it and using it to plan improvements (organizations without Internet access may request a hard copy;

however, cumulative reporting features are available online only).

The PEPNet Results Assessment Tool (with Benchmarking Capability) captures and organizes youth performance data, allowing users to compare actual performance with program goals as well as with the performance of programs around the country. Users select the outcomes and progress measures that a program tracks and enter corresponding performance data. From that information, the tool generates a results analysis report with numerical information and descriptive text about the program's result. For select PEPNet outcomes, the tool also provides benchmarks, comparing results to a national group of programs serving youth of similar populations and localities.

The PEPNet Improvement Action Planning Tool enables the user to review areas for improvement already identified through the Self Assessment or Results Assessment tools described above. The user can then translate these into improvement goals and create an action plan. The tool walks the user through prioritizing areas for improvement, setting goals, identifying strategies to achieve goals, and defining action steps, responsible parties, and needed resources. Users may revisit the plan to review or edit record actions taken and eventually mark the goal as completed.

NYEC EDNet is a tool for continuous improvement for education programs and schools serving vulnerable youth. It consists of detailed criteria identified as common to effective education programs and schools by a national working group of educators, practitioners, policymakers, and researchers and a comprehensive self-assessment that can assist education programs and schools in improving their services and also inform policymakers, funders, and the public about what works for youth.

Notes

1. Sum, A., Khatiwada, I., McLaughlin, J., & Palma, S. (2005). *The paradox of rising teen joblessness in an expanding labor market: The absence of teen employment growth in the national jobs recovery of 2003–2004.* Boston: Northeastern University, Center for Labor Market Studies.

2. Swanson, C. (2004). *Who graduates? Who doesn't? A statistical portrait of public high school graduation, class of 2001.* Washington, DC: Urban Institute.

NEW DIRECTIONS FOR YOUTH DEVELOPMENT • DOI: 10.1002/yd

3. Gunderson, S. (2004, January). *The fifth revolution: America's emerging workforce.* PowerPoint presentation to the U.S. Conference of Mayors, Boston.

4. Sum et al. (2005).

5. Comprehensive Employment and Training Act of 1973, Public Law 93–203, et seq., 87 Stat. 839.

6. Zuckerman, A. (2000). The more things change, the more they stay the same: The evolution and devolution of youth employment programs. In N. Jaffe (Ed.), *Youth development: Issues, challenges and direction* (pp. 301–324). Philadelphia: Public/Private Ventures.

7. Walker, K. (1997). *Some things do make a difference for youth: A compendium of evaluations of youth programs and practices.* Washington, DC: American Youth Policy Forum.

8. Workforce Investment Act of 1998, Public Law 105–220—Aug. 7, 1998, 112 Stat. 936.

9. Brown, D. (1998). Advancing youth development under the Workforce Investment Act. *Workforce Investment Quarterly, 5*(4), 45.

10. The NYEC is a national membership network of over 285 member organizations in forty-one states dedicated to improving the effectiveness of organizations that seek to help youth become productive citizens. NYEC strives to achieve its mission by tracking, crafting, and influencing policy; setting and promoting standards; promoting professional development; and building the organizational capacity of youth-serving organizations. Its diverse membership includes a broad-based constituency of direct service providers, local and state education and workforce agencies, research and policy organizations, national organizations, and technical assistance providers. The majority of NYEC's membership is focused on improving policies and practices for youth aged fourteen to twenty-five who have been poorly served by traditional youth-serving systems and are least likely to make a successful transition to adulthood.

11. To ensure that the PEPNet standards are current, NYEC has embarked on the PEPNet Enhancement Project. It has received comments from practitioners, researchers, policymakers, and funders from across the nation and is conducting an extensive literature review on what young people need to know and be able to do. NYEC is also engaged in a review of empirical studies on youth programs and practices that have been effective in helping young people achieve positive outcomes.

12. NYEC is preparing to release the Guide to Measuring and Documenting Youth Program Outcomes to help programs, funders, and policymakers work on this challenging area; understand PEPNet's outcomes and progress measures; and improve measurement.

13. National Collaborative on Workforce and Disability for Youth. (2002). *Literature review: Frontline worker. What's missing?* Retrieved March 4, 2004, from www.ncwdyouth.info/assets/literature_Reviews/frontline_worker_summary.pdf; Goodwill Industries International. (2002). *Strategies for developing a 21st century youth services initiative.* Bethesda, MD: Goodwill Industries International; Pearson, S. (2001). *Preparing youth with disabilities for an increasingly technical work place.* Briefing from Capital Hill Forum, January 26, 2001.

Washington, DC: American Youth Policy Forum. Retrieved March 4, 2004, from www.aypf.org/subcats/ydlist.htm.

14. National Collaborative on Workforce and Disability for Youth. (2002); Goodwill Industries International. (2002); Pearson. (2001).

DAVID E. BROWN *is the deputy director of the District of Columbia's Department of Youth Rehabilitation Services.*

MALA B. THAKUR *serves as the acting executive director of the National Youth Employment Coalition.*

Communities that want to build a system of supports to meet the unique developmental and programmatic needs of the older youth population must do so in the context of a communitywide strategy as opposed to fragmented, individually operating programs and services.

8

Going the distance: Serving the needs of older youth at scale

Mark Ouellette

FEW COMMUNITIES HAVE DEVELOPED successful strategies for attracting large numbers of older youth to their out-of-school-time programs. Older youth are a challenging population to serve programmatically for several reasons:

- Demanding schedules mean that young people's participation on a regular basis can be challenging.
- Teens are not necessarily motivated to seek out positive programming alternatives because they enjoy simply hanging out with peers.
- Many programs stop focusing on young people because they struggle with sustaining their interest and involvement over time.
- Many programs are not flexible enough to adapt to the growing autonomy and changing interests of teens to successfully provide them with supports and opportunities that can help them through the challenges of adolescence.

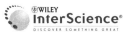

NEW DIRECTIONS FOR YOUTH DEVELOPMENT, NO. 111, FALL 2006 © WILEY PERIODICALS, INC.
Published online in Wiley InterScience (www.interscience.wiley.com) • DOI: 10.1002/yd.186

105

- Although many high schools offer a range of extracurricular activities, they tend to attract students who are at least moderately engaged in school. There are few opportunities for teens who are not engaged in school.
- Preparing teens for the world of work and higher education and addressing risk factors may require special programming and staff sensitive to these needs.

In addition to meeting the unique programmatic needs of the older youth population, communities have struggled with the challenge of creating communitywide integrated approaches to service delivery and resource development. This chapter explores the rationale for creating and implementing communitywide older youth support approaches and offers concrete recommendations for planning and action.

Why should communities care?

The United States has a growing number of disconnected youth. Among the 2.9 million large-city residents aged sixteen to twenty-four who were not enrolled in school, more than 1 million did not work. This means that more than 18 percent of the sixteen- to twenty-four-year-old population in these large cities was disconnected from both school and work and not on a pathway toward high school completion.[1]

The following statistics, gathered by Henry Levin, professor of economics and education at Teachers College, Columbia University, suggest the impact that out-of-school youth have on society, such as huge public costs in crime, welfare assistance, health care, and lost taxes:

- Adults without a high school diploma are twice as likely to be unemployed.
- They will earn $260,000 less over a lifetime than a high school graduate.

- Dropouts make up nearly 70 percent of inmates crowding state prisons and at least half of those on welfare.
- Their life expectancy is 9.2 years lower than that of high school graduates.
- The average forty-five-year-old dropout is in worse health than the average sixty-five-year-old high school graduate.[2]

Expanding services to older youth

Many communities' out-of-school-time programs and services target children at the elementary school level. Once students enter middle school, they are much less likely to participate in after-school and community programs, and their participation drops even further when they enter high school. Knowing this, many communities look at out-of-school-time programs as an extension of day care until children are old enough to look after themselves unsupervised. Nevertheless, the need for out-of-school-time supports and opportunities does not disappear with age.

Older students are expected to master several academic, social, and developmental benchmarks as they face key transitions from elementary to middle school and middle school to high school. By developing opportunities for older youth, communities can provide an avenue for helping them successfully navigate these key developmental challenges. Such programs must be age and developmentally appropriate, challenging, culturally relevant, and connected to the students' daily lives.

Quality out-of-school-time programming for older youth often focuses on students' psychosocial development by striving to foster an age-appropriate sense of independence and develop students' ability to resist risky behaviors. Also, many of these programs aim to facilitate positive youth development by providing high school students with separate environments, where they can explore new skill areas, engage in problem solving and decision making, discover talents within themselves, and develop positive relationships with adults and peers. Programs designed to foster youth development build on the assets and strengths of young people, recognizing their needs for both ongoing support and challenging opportunities. These initiatives are in contrast to programs that simply attempt to "fix" adolescents by addressing only problem behaviors such as school dropout, early pregnancy, or substance abuse.

Communities wanting to build a system of supports for older youth must do so in the context of a communitywide strategy as opposed to fragmented, individually operating programs and services. A communitywide strategy creates greater opportunity for strategic mobilization of resources, greater funding leverage, evaluation and assessment consistency, and more powerful input into creating a public voice and public will for supporting and serving older youth.

Elements of going the distance

Innovative communitywide strategies to meet the needs of older youth are starting to emerge. We have learned a fair amount from initiatives such as Chicago's After School Matters, and can glean that in order to go to scale, the following five system-level components are essential:

- An understanding of what youth want in out-of-school-time programs
- Communitywide leadership with an effective plan
- Coordination among key stakeholders
- High school programming standards that include youth voice
- Coordinated and adequate funding

An understanding of what youth want in out-of-school-time programs

With today's emphasis on raising standards and reducing dropout rates, some educators, policy makers, and parents want to use more out-of-school time to ramp up learning for both youngsters in danger of failing and those who want to get an edge on college admissions. The benefits of these academic pursuits might seem obvious to adults, but it is hardly surprising that most youth do not view them so favorably. On a national survey, 61 percent indicate that "when the school day is done, the last thing I want is to go to a place that has more academic work." Even so, some youth report that they would very much like an after-school program that provides homework help or focuses on academics. Given a choice among organized activities that emphasize sports, the arts, or academics, 9 percent of youth favor academic preparation, 54 percent choose sports, and 36 percent choose something "like art, music, or dance." More than half of the students surveyed acknowledge that they could use extra help in some subjects (55 percent) and express an interest in summer programs that would help them keep up with schoolwork or prepare for the next grade (56 percent).[3]

Communitywide leadership with an effective plan

With the myriad of potential providers of out-of-school-time programs for older youth, a community that wants to go the distance needs a local champion to carry the initiative. This can be a municipal leader, a school superintendent, business leader, or other well-respected champion. Mayors are natural leaders, as they are representatives of an entire city. Following are examples of how municipal leaders used their influence and office to develop a system of opportunity and programming for older youth.

In his 2002 State of City Address, Mayor Richard M. Daley of Chicago stated the city goal is to "provide [every year] more high-quality after-school and summer programs so that more of our children can participate in meaningful alternatives that engage them and keep them away from gangs, guns, and drugs." The expansion of after-school programs is not just a vision but an official priority of the mayor.[4]

Mayor Anthony A. Williams of Washington, D.C., and his staff conducted research and identified a youth development approach for framing all of its programs. Youth development is the ongoing growth process in which all youth are engaged in attempting to meet their personal and social needs to be safe, feel cared for, be valued, be useful, be spiritually grounded, and build skills and competencies that allow them to function and contribute in their daily lives.

NEW DIRECTIONS FOR YOUTH DEVELOPMENT • DOI: 10.1002/yd

As a result of this research, Mayor Williams has developed the Effective Youth Development Plan, and all programs for youth, from juvenile justice to school success, are measured against this document. In the document, Williams states,

Youth development is happening whether adults and institutions are around or not. As they grow, young people will seek out ways to get [their] needs met. It is our societal responsibility to provide the appropriate services, supports and opportunities to young people so that this process can be a positive one. Using the Search Institute's nationally recognized '40 Developmental Assets' framework, positive, healthy development for all young people regardless of socio-economic status, geography or ethnicity can be measured in the presence of support, empowerment, boundaries and expectations, constructive uses of time, commitment of learning, positive values, social competencies, and positive identity.[5]

Many cities have created an office of youth development to oversee all of these different agencies. The purpose is typically to expand opportunities, support, and services to youth throughout the community by (1) expanding opportunities for youth to participate in decision making; (2) increasing opportunities for internships, volunteer service, and mentorship; (3) increasing coordination among youth-serving organizations; and (4) providing community education about youth development and the developmental asset framework.

In New York City, Mayor Rudy Giuliani and, after him, Mayor Michael Bloomberg, have spent the past ten years reestablishing and enhancing the Department of Youth and Community Development (DYCD) as an integration of two separate agencies, the Department of Youth Services and the Community Development Agency. This merger took place in October 1996.

A single structure that incorporates the core mission of both of these agencies to strengthen community resources and provide services to many of the same youth and low-income populations was created to oversee the contracts formerly administered by the two agencies without eliminating any existing programs or reducing service levels. Through this consolidation, DYCD became the lead agency for providing comprehensive services to youth, families, and their communities. The consolidation became a resourceful and creative way to maintain service delivery during a tough fiscal period. Because social service agencies often provided overlapping services and interacted with many of the same clients, consolidating their functions eliminated duplication, created efficiencies, improved program operations, and conserved funds.

During 2003, Mayor Bloomberg signed legislation to streamline social service programs by eliminating the Department of Employment and relocating youth employment programs and services to DYCD. Situating youth programs in a single agency gave DYCD the opportunity to coordinate a broader range of youth development initiatives. The consolidation offered a commonsense approach to the delivery of human services, which ultimately improved client access.

Coordination among key stakeholders

Another strategy for developing municipal leadership is the creation of an office of youth development as a cabinet-level position. In many cities, a variety of agencies and organizations provide services to young people. In the District of Columbia, over eighteen government agencies provide programming or funding for older youth, and communication and coordination among agencies is challenging. Establishing a coordinating role at a high level in local government can establish a consistent framework for program and service providers to synchronize their mutual efforts to support older youth.

Building partnerships within the community strengthens youth programming, an important component of the community, and the community can provide an abundance of resources to enrich program quality. By developing positive relationships with agencies and businesses and engaging in joint activities, programs can offer older youth ample opportunities for internships, career exploration and training, and opportunities to develop community spirit and good citizenship skills.

After School Matters in Chicago is an example of a successful coordination model. To build the type of program that Mayor and

Maggie Daley envisioned, youth would have to move freely from the school system, to the libraries, and the parks system. For this to happen, Mayor Daly had several high-ranking aides address turf issues and barriers. The program also has been highly successful in coordinating funding between public and private resources.

Program standards that include youth voice

In 2002, the National Research Council released *Community Programs to Promote Youth Development*, which greatly contributed to our understanding of the field of youth development.[6] In this publication, an advisory council of national experts identified a set of personal and social assets that increase the healthy development and well-being of adolescents and facilitate a successful transition from childhood through adolescence, and into adulthood. These assets were grouped into four broad developmental domains: physical, intellectual, psychological and emotional, and social development. While communities consider these recommendations, we also know that the most critical factor contributing to the success or failure of older youth programming is whether young people find it appealing. Program designers must make a number of decisions about design and operation, including matching activities to participants' needs, using resources effectively, and recruiting participants.

One important element is that programming should be dynamic and responsive to participants' needs. One high school program responded to student interest in rock climbing by combining lessons with other outdoor programming. Some students want independent study alternatives to classes; some want programs that focus on recreation or community involvement. An increase in grants or donations may extend program hours; cutbacks may result in reduced activity selection. Programming can and should change as circumstances change.

For more than three years, youth in Columbus, Ohio, have made their opinions heard through the Columbus Youth Commission (CYC), an advisory group formed in collaboration with the Columbus City Council and Mayor Michael B. Coleman, a member of the National League of Cities' Council on Youth, Education, and Fam-

NEW DIRECTIONS FOR YOUTH DEVELOPMENT • DOI: 10.1002/yd

ilies. Twenty-one teens and young adults aged thirteen to twenty-one participate. The mission of the CYC is to provide leadership in the development of priorities and a comprehensive agenda for youth. This includes:

- Developing recommendations and solutions for youth issues
- Linking youth initiatives and programming to enhance service, increase awareness, and promote the efficient use of resources
- Developing, organizing, and hosting the annual Youth Summit
- Developing methods to measure the overall results and impact of the commission
- Providing an annual report to the mayor and city council regarding youth programming in the Columbus area

Columbus Youth Commission chair Tei Street states, "The city is committed to serving all of its citizens, and we can't do that if everyone's voice is not represented. Young people should be at the table to give adults guidance and feedback in addressing and redressing their own issues."[7]

Coordinated and adequate funding

One of the largest challenges for building a communitywide strategy is finding adequate funding for programs and services for older youth. More than likely, a combination of federal, state, city, and private dollars is needed. One way to begin the process in the community is to ask these five questions:

- What is the current investment in older youth programs and services?
- What is the need for older youth programs and services in our community?
- How much do we expect to spend per youth on programs and services?
- How will the community address the gap?
- How will the community leverage the public's investment?

NEW DIRECTIONS FOR YOUTH DEVELOPMENT • DOI: 10.1002/yd

Sustainability will require creative and flexible financing. Houston's After School Achievement Program (ASAP) began in 1997 with a budget of $140,000 and has expanded to a budget of $3.2 million, serving twelve thousand youth. The program's revenues come from four primary sources: city general fund revenues, a Community Development Block Grant, the Housing Resolution Trust (Housing), and, recently, state juvenile justice funds.

ASAP is also implementing a new strategy for ASAP programs to become self-sufficient. This shift will free up city funds to sponsor more programs and expand. In the first year, sites are eligible for up to forty thousand dollars and are required to provide only an in-kind match of ten thousand dollars. During the second year, sites may receive up to thirty thousand dollars and must match with ten thousand dollars in cash and ten thousand dollars in kind. Third-, fourth-, and fifth-year sites are eligible for twenty thousand dollars and must match with twenty thousand dollars in cash and ten thousand dollars in-kind.

Conclusion

Going to scale on providing programs and services for older youth is challenging but needed. It takes a considerable amount of thinking, coordination, planning, funding, and training. The reward is significant: older youth are provided with meaningful opportunities that facilitate a smooth and healthy transition into adulthood.

Notes

1. Sum, A., Khatiwada, I., McLaughlin, J., & Palma, S. (2005). *The paradox of rising teen joblessness in an expanding labor market: The absence of teen employment growth in the national jobs recovery of 2003–2004.* Boston: Northeastern University, Center for Labor Market Studies.

2. Peterson, K. (2006, January 11). *Education quandary: Curbing dropouts.* Retrieved from http://www. stateline.org/live/ViewPage.action?site NodeId=136&languageId=1&contentId=79589.

3. Duffett, A., Johnson, J., Farkas, S., Kung, S., & Ott, A. (2004). *All work and no play? Listening to what kids and parents really want from out-of-school time.* New York: Public Agenda.

4. Proscio, T. (2002). *Precious time: A report to the field.* New York: After School Project.

5. District of Columbia. (2005). *Effective youth development: A strategy to ensure district youth grow-up problem free, fully prepared and fully engaged.* Washington, DC: Author.

6. National Research Council and Institute of Medicine. (2002). *Community programs to promote youth development.* Washington, DC: National Academy Press.

7. Haehle, H. (2005). *Columbus, Ohio listens to youth.* Washington, DC: National League of Cities, Nation's Cities Weekly. Retrieved October 2, 2006, from http://www.nlc.org/Newsroom/ Nation_s_Cities_Weekly/ Weekly_NCW/2005/11/28/7204.cfm.

MARK OUELLETTE *is the director of programs and policy at the District of Columbia Children and Youth Investment Trust Corporation.*

State and local policy innovations that promote increased investments in institutions, community programs, and youth services are developing across the country and can inform out-of-school-time strategies for older youth.

9

Supporting older youth: What's policy got to do with it?

Nicole Yohalem, Alicia Wilson-Ahlstrom, Thaddeus Ferber, Elizabeth Gaines

WITH THE EDUCATION SPOTLIGHT shifting to secondary schools and conversations about dropout rates, high school redesign, and workforce readiness taking place in government agencies, schools, universities, businesses, and foundations across the country, teenagers have become a focus of serious policy discussion. It is imperative that the evolving conversation not simply consider school reform or the challenges presented by teens' nonschool hours. Too often we respond to youth issues with fragmented and disjointed responses, lacking a clear plan for promoting positive outcomes. The policy conversation should be about—and in some states and communities it increasingly is about—what it will take for young people to be ready for college, ready for work, and ready for life.

The good news is that pockets of innovation are developing in districts, communities, and states across the country as ambitious

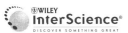

public and private agencies and creative individuals push the envelope in terms of where, when, and how teens learn and develop. Noteworthy policy examples are emerging at the administrative/ regulatory and legislative levels, informing the design and implementation of services as well as broader policy initiatives and mandates. This chapter begins at the service delivery level, highlighting specific policy innovations related to teens' involvement in out-of-school-time activities. We then broaden our lens to look at three principles we believe can help ensure that youth policy supports the full range of older youth's developmental, social, and economic needs.

Maximizing out-of-school-time for older youth

The nonschool hours are an underused tool in supporting older youth in their transition to adulthood. High-quality programs can help young people become ready for college, work, and life, but such opportunities decline with age, and older youth participation is inconsistent.[1] Given competing demands on many teens' time and a host of other developmental realities, effective strategies for engaging high schoolers look much different than they do for their younger counterparts, and those differences have both programmatic and policy implications.[2]

We have chosen to highlight five issues that demonstrate how policies related to out-of-school time can be aligned with the developmental needs of older youth: financial incentives, school credit, alternative pathways to credentials, participation requirements, and funding. We then broaden our discussion beyond administrative and regulatory policies that inform program implementation and beyond out-of-school time to discuss several principles we believe can help guide youth policy development at all levels and on a range of issues.

Financial incentives

Idleness is not the norm for teenagers in the afternoon. Many teens, particularly those from low-income families, have no choice but to work or take on family responsibilities after school. At the same time,

NEW DIRECTIONS FOR YOUTH DEVELOPMENT • DOI: 10.1002/yd

employment opportunities for low-income teens are on the decline. Between 2000 and 2003, the annual average number of employed sixteen to twenty-four year olds declined by nearly 1.1 million, or 5.2 percent, far exceeding employment declines for all other age groups.[3] While some work is considered healthy for this age group, studies suggest that working twenty hours per week or more is linked to sleep loss, reduced school performance, and health risks.[4] Programs that provide young people with career development opportunities through internships, job shadowing, employment training, and on-the-job experience can address two important developmental tasks simultaneously: preparing young people for adulthood and the world of work and compensating them for their time.

After School Matters (ASM) is a citywide partnership between the City of Chicago, the Chicago Public Schools, the Chicago Park District, the Chicago Public Library, and the Chicago Department of Children and Youth Services. Through this partnership, ASM provides three-day-a-week paid apprenticeships to over four thousand high school youth in a number of creative and professional disciplines. Apprenticeships, led primarily by adult professionals working in each discipline, are intentionally designed to lead to summer or even longer-term employment. In addition to providing stipends, ASM offers real-world experiences and environments, access to mentors who are experts in an area of interest, and a schedule that appropriately accommodates the realities of teenagers' weekly responsibilities and commitments.

The After-School Corporation (TASC) in New York has developed an academic support and career development program using Workforce Investment Act (WIA) funds to target high school students at risk of dropping out of school. The program engages cohorts of teens during the after-school hours and the summer in activities geared toward academic achievement, career planning, and work experience. Participants receive stipends for internships around the city at places like the Metropolitan Museum of Art, Mt. Sinai Hospital, the United Nations, and local middle and elementary schools. They are supported by fellowship advisers in their high schools who use a case manager approach to advise on career planning and academic improvement and help coordinate and maximize teens' school and out-of-school activities.

These programs and others that provide financial incentives to participating youth have done so by blending funding streams and building creative partnerships with the business community and other agencies. Placing a greater emphasis on career development in out-of-school-time programs and ensuring flexibility in how funds are spent will help more programs compensate young people for their time. This move is both developmentally appropriate and strategic if we hope to offer compelling after-school options for older youth.

School credit

Teens want to develop skills and participate in opportunities that support their goals for the future by helping them understand, prepare for, and navigate their post–high school options. And they want their nonschool hours to count toward these goals.[5] While many school districts around the country have put in place community service requirements and allow students to fulfill them through community-based activities, after-school programs are rarely considered formal learning environments where academic credit can be earned. There are some exceptions, however, where community-based resources are being brought to bear on formal learning in concrete ways.

Camdenton, Missouri, has used 21st Century Community Learning Center (21st CCLC) funds to launch an extended-hours program called Credit Recovery that enables high school students who have failed one core subject to regain credit in that subject and get back on track toward graduation. Students work with certified teachers who use a range of support strategies, including discussion groups and individual tutoring instruction. The course work is self-paced, individualized, and intentionally designed to align with core curriculum courses.

Educational Video Center helps New York City public high school students earn school credit each year through its semester-long after-school Documentary Workshop. Students learn to shoot and edit documentaries on issues important to their lives as urban teens, and in the process, they develop skills in media analysis, script writing, interviewing, editing, camera work, and video documentary production using state-of-the-art equipment. At the end of each semester, students present their work in public screenings and are assessed in portfolio roundtables. The tapes and viewer guides are then made available for public distribution.

These two examples and others around the country, where students earn credits for work accomplished outside the school day and school building, are possible only through strong partnerships between schools and out-of-school-time providers. Creative leaders in the school and after-school settings are working together to identify and overcome potential administrative obstacles, discuss student needs, and align curricula. These kinds of relationships can be facilitated or discouraged based on the accessibility and flexibility of funding opportunities and the graduation expectations and mandates of the school system.

Alternative pathways to credentials

Relatively isolated policy discussions have taken place over the past decade about the idea of competency- or proficiency-based assessment. However, with the spotlight on high school dropout rates and employer concerns about workforce readiness on the rise, these discussions are likely to move into the mainstream. As they do, the full range of school- and community-based learning environments where young people spend time should be part of the conversation, particularly if, in order to graduate, students must demonstrate mastery of both academic subject matter and skills like teamwork, communication, and cultural competence. Research about adolescent time use suggests that youth in voluntary out-of-school-time programs report very high levels of both concentration and motivation compared with other places they spend time.[6] These settings should be taken seriously as additional contexts for learning and for developing and demonstrating mastery.

Oregon has had in place since 1993 the Proficiency-Based Admissions Standards System (PASS), an effort to align the K–12 education system with university admissions by awarding certificates of mastery to high school students that both help them graduate and contribute toward the college admissions process. In 2002, the state board of education approved a proficiency-based credit system, where districts can award diploma credits based on the satisfactory completion of work that takes place in an alternative program, which may include career-related experiences and project-based learning that takes place outside the school day or school building.[7]

The U.S. Chamber of Commerce, along with several states, cities, and other national partners like the National Urban League and the National Association of Manufacturing, are working together to promote the Equipped for the Future Workforce Readiness Credential, intended to become a national credential to assess whether young people have a solid foundation in the skills and abilities they will need to succeed in the workplace. The credential would be voluntary and portable across states and is not intended to compete with the high school diploma. Earning a credential would require successfully demonstrating a range of interpersonal, decision-making, and communication skills—skills that many out-of-school-time programs are well positioned to help students develop.[8]

While Oregon's PASS program remains unique and a national credential like the one described would take years to implement and presents a range of complex policy challenges, discussions about competency-based assessment are increasing, as is the urgency to do something to address the fact that too few young people leave high school ready for work, college, and life. The full range of learning environments where young people spend time warrants close consideration in a competency-based system, where what matters is whether students master skills, not where they develop them.

Participation requirements

By high school, most teens have some degree of freedom to manage their schedules, and many have increased family and work responsibilities. This increased discretion means they are likely to be more selective about when and where they choose to participate in voluntary activities, which has important implications for scheduling and attendance requirements. Funding and other administrative regulations should reflect the real participation patterns of teens and the need for greater flexibility.

NEW DIRECTIONS FOR YOUTH DEVELOPMENT • DOI: 10.1002/yd

The After-School Corporation (TASC) allows teens to check in with after-school program staff on days they are attending an internship with a local employer and still be recognized as participating in an after-school activity. This strategy honors the fact that teens are using their time constructively and facilitates regular connections between teens and staff liaisons who play a case manager role, connecting school and after-school activities and advising students on college and career planning.

The California Department of Education created tiered participation targets for 21st CCLC-funded high school programs that link with different levels of expected outcomes. So rather than expect all participants to attend programs four or five times a week, as is required of elementary programs, high school programs are asked to set targets for engaging a certain percentage of teens for whom program expectations are higher and who therefore will attend frequently, another percentage who will attend less frequently and for whom expectations are adjusted, and so on.

Opening the doors to programs does not guarantee student participation, particularly when it comes to older youth and those at risk for school failure. Attendance-based funding regulations should take into account developmental differences in participation, and checks and balances should be put in place so that programs are not incentivized to recruit less vulnerable or younger participants who are likely to attend programs more frequently.

Funding

Efforts to substantially expand out-of-school time opportunities for older youth face a basic policy challenge in that existing funding streams disproportionately support younger children. The largest federal funding stream, the Child Care Development Block Grant, covers only low-income children ages twelve and younger.[9] Proposition 49 in California will infuse over $500 million into elementary and middle school programming. While Department of Education 21st CCLC funds can be used to support programs at elementary, middle, and high schools, only 6 percent of currently funded centers serve high school students.[10]

While this disparity likely stems in part from local programs deciding how to target limited resources, it may also be explained by a legislative requirement that at least 40 percent of students in participating schools be eligible for free or reduced-price lunch. Because of their size and broader geographical reach, far fewer high schools meet this threshold than elementary or middle schools. While states can apply for a waiver or set priorities for serving certain populations, this requirement is likely part of the reason that so few high schools receive these funds. Despite regulatory and other challenges, the following examples show how public and private agencies are finding creative ways to secure funding for high school after-school programming.

California put in place a formal legislative set-aside in 2002 to ensure funding would be available for high school programs. As a result, the legislation funded sixteen after-school programs beginning in 2003 using federal 21st CLCC dollars. In addition to setting aside funds for this age group, the legislation called for a commitment to capacity-building support so that this effort would be sure to yield important lessons about the unique programming needs of high school students.[11]

Philadelphia Youth Network (PYN) is a workforce development intermediary that contracts federal Workforce Investment Act dollars out to twenty-six different youth organizations around the city that serve over four thousand youth annually through after-school and summer career development programs. The logistical challenges of applying for WIA funds and complying with federal regulations mean that intermediaries like PYN (and TASC, discussed earlier) can play an important role in helping individual after-school programs access and successfully use these dollars.

A commitment to funding high school afterschool could help bridge gaps among multiple funding streams. Unlike most funding for youth programs, created in response to specific problems (for example, gang diversion, pregnancy prevention, or employment training), after-school funding is framed around a specific period of time. By approaching young people's lives by time of day rather than depth of problem, mandates for high school afterschool could be used to tap both after-school and other sources like the WIA.

Principles for effective youth policies

While focused efforts to increase the quality and quantity of out-of-school-time opportunities for older youth are important, it is equally important that out-of-school time not be considered an isolated policy issue.[12] The fundamental goal behind this and other important yet often disconnected conversations is to better prepare young people for productive futures by ensuring they make the transition to adulthood ready to meet the demands. Effective youth policies reflect an overarching vision that is about changing lives: a vision that addresses a range of risk and protective factors, simultaneously supports discrete programs and builds coherent pathways to success, and recognizes that children and youth grow up in families and communities.[13] The following principles and examples illustrate how states and communities are working to make supports for children and youth more effective, accessible, and connected to families and communities.

Focus on youth's strengths and assets, not just discrete problems

Traditionally, public officials have approached youth policy by tackling one problem at a time: youth violence one year, juvenile delinquency another, substance abuse the next. While we have become quite sophisticated at measuring and in some cases preventing the behaviors we want youth to avoid, most states and localities are not in the habit of measuring and promoting behaviors we know will help them prepare for successful futures. There are, however, some exceptions worth noting.

Louisiana, Maine, and some other states are setting positive developmental results or goals for young people that cut across academic, social, and physical well-being. Many states are also finding ways to track positive development, allowing policymakers and the public to base decisions on what it is they want to see, as opposed to what they want to avoid. In Vermont, state agencies are part of a public-private partnership to develop, disseminate, and use data on positive indicators; their framework includes outcomes of well-being, positive social indicators, measurement tools, legislation, and community-based data collection strategies.[14]

Build comprehensive, coordinated efforts that cross traditional lines

A survey of state legislators found that building a coherent message on children's policy is challenging "because there is no clearly discernible legislative agenda for children and families; rather, a multitude of individuals and organizations with different agendas are sending mixed messages about what is best for children."[15] With legislatures organized into committees and executive branches into departments, each responsible for different policies and programs, policymakers are forced to make decisions that may not reflect a clear understanding of the nature of the problem or a complete view of relevant initiatives already under way. This challenge is compounded by fragmentation within the advocacy community, which tends to be organized around specific issues and policies. Weaving the existing tangle of services into a seamless web of supports requires working across issues as well as departmental, committee, and sometimes partisan lines.

In response to this challenge, many states are building children's cabinets, joint legislative committees, or other structures to improve coordination and communication, and many are using tools like youth budgets and report cards to illustrate their investments and progress across a range of programs and outcome areas. The Louisiana Children's Cabinet, for example, was created by the legislature in 1998 and includes secretaries from several relevant departments (including education, social services, and public safety), a senator, a representative, and members of the state's supreme court and board of education. The group produces a children's budget each year and works across its membership to improve and coordinate services. Maryland's Joint Committee on Children, Youth and Families is charged with recommending new laws, regulations, and budget priorities to improve children's well-being. It also searches out and makes recommendations to remedy interdepartmental gaps, inconsistencies, or inefficiencies in children and youth services and informs the legislature and public on relevant issues.[16]

Bring youth perspectives to the table

"If you had a problem in the black community, and you brought together a group of white people to discuss how to solve it, almost nobody would take that panel seriously. In fact there'd probably be a public outcry. But every day, in local arenas all the way to the White House, adults sit around and decide what problems youth have and what youth need, without ever consulting us."[17] This seventeen year old articulates a critical challenge facing policymakers charged with making decisions that affect the lives of a largely non-voting constituency. While it is relatively easy to bring in a single young person to consult on a policy decision, involving large numbers of youth is difficult. Training and support are needed so that young people are well versed on the issues and the policymaking process and so that the adults are prepared to fully engage and work in partnership with the young people.

In addition to investing in civic education to encourage lifelong civic involvement and create avenues for youth to share their perspectives, many states and localities have created youth councils or other advisory bodies designed to create meaningful roles for youth in shaping policies that affect them. Youth members of Maine's Legislative Youth Advisory Council, for example, conduct public hearings, draft bills, and make recommendations on proposals that are under consideration by the legislature. In 2003, New Mexico's legislature created the New Mexico Youth Alliance, which consists of 112 youth from across the state, to advise the governor, lieutenant governor, and legislature on youth policy issues. Recruiting young people who reflect the diversity of the state or community in question is an important consideration, as is providing the resources and infrastructure necessary for these kinds of groups to be more than symbolic.

New public ideas

While being intentional about all of these principles and building a holistic policy approach to supporting older youth may seem unrealistic and challenging to take to scale, entertaining alternative public ideas about what is possible is a hallmark of an effective democracy. According to Moore, the core responsibility of those who deal in public policy "is not simply to discover as objectively as possible what people want for themselves and then to determine and implement the best means of satisfying those wants. It is also to provide the public with alternative visions of what is desirable and possible, to stimulate deliberation about them, provoke a reexamination of premises and values, and thus to broaden the range of potential responses and deepen society's understanding of itself."[18]

It is only when we effectively engage the full range of stakeholders committed to supporting children and youth that we will develop ideas that will go beyond the status quo. Preparing young people for the future requires more than improving high schools or expanding out-of-school-time opportunities; it requires the full engagement of all community institutions, small and large, public and private, in supporting learning and development.

Notes

1. Tolman, J., Pittman, K., Yohalem, N., Thomases, J., & Trammel, M. (2002). *Moving an out-of-school agenda: Lessons and challenges across cities.* Washington, DC: Forum for Youth Investment.

2. Forum for Youth Investment. (2003). *Out-of-school-time policy commentary #5: Inside the black box: What is the "content" of after-school?* Washington, DC: Forum for Youth Investment, Impact Strategies. Retrieved November 1, 2005, from www.forumfyi.org/Files//ostpc5.pdf.

3. Sum, A. & Khatiwada, I. (2004). *Still young, restless, and jobless: The growing employment malaise among U.S. teens and young adults.* Alexandria, VA: Jobs for America's Graduates. Retrieved November 1, 2005, from www.nyec.org/CLS&JAG_report.pdf.

4. Lerman, R. I. (2000). *Are teens in low-income and welfare families working too much? Number B-25 in New Federalism: National Survey of America's Families.* Retrieved November 2005 from http://newfederalism.urban.org/html/series_b/anf_b25.html.

5. Hall, G., Israel, L., & Shortt, J. (2004). *It's about time: A look at out-of-school time for urban teens.* Wellesley, MA: National Institute on Out-of-School Time. Retrieved November 1, 2005, from www.niost.org/AOLTW.pdf.

6. Larson, R. (2000). Toward a psychology of positive youth development. *American Psychologist, 55*(1), 170–183.

7. Thakur, M., & Henry, K. (2005). *Financing alternative education pathways: Profiles and policy.* Washington, DC: National Youth Employment Coalition.

8. Forum for Youth Investment. (2003).

9. Finance Project. (2004, October). *CCDF and 21CCLC state efforts to facilitate coordination for afterschool programs.* Washington, DC: Child Care Bureau of the U.S. Department of Health and Human Services. Retrieved November 1, 2005, from www.financeproject.org/Publications/CCDF%20_21CCLC.pdf.

10. Forum for Youth Investment. (2005). *Out-of-school-time policy commentary #10: Rethinking the high school experience: What's after-school got to do with it?* Washington, DC: Forum for Youth Investment, Impact Strategies. Retrieved November 1, 2005, from www.forumfyi.org/Files/ostpc10.pdf.

11. Forum for Youth Investment (2004a). *High school: The next frontier for after-school advocates?* Washington, DC: Forum for Youth Investment, Impact Strategies. Retrieved November 1, 2005, from www.forumfyi.org/Files//ForumFOCUS_Feb2004.pdf.

12. Wright, E. (2005). *Supporting student success: A governor's guide to extra learning opportunities.* Washington, DC: National Governors Association Center for Best Practices.

13. Ferber, T., Gaines, E., & Goodman, C. (2005). *Positive youth development: State strategies. Strengthening youth policy research and policy report.* Denver: National Conference of State Legislatures. Retrieved January 20, 2006, from http://www.forumfyi.org/Files//strengtheningyouthpolicy.pdf.

14. Forum for Youth Investment. (2004b). *What gets measured gets done.* Washington, DC: Forum for Youth Investment, Impact Strategies.

15. State Legislative Leaders Foundation. (1995). *State legislative leaders: Keys to effective legislation for children and families.* Centerville, MA: State Legislative Leaders Foundation.

16. Ferber et al. (2005).

17 Ferber et al. (2005).

18. Moore, M. (1998). What sort of ideas become public ideas? In R. Reich (Ed.), *The power of public ideas.* Cambridge, MA: Harvard University Press.

NICOLE YOHALEM *is a program director at the Forum for Youth Investment.*

ALICIA WILSON-AHLSTROM *is a program manager at the Forum for Youth Investment.*

THADDEUS FERBER *is a program director at the Forum for Youth Investment.*

ELIZABETH GAINES *is a program manager at the Forum for Youth Investment.*

Index

Back Issue/Subscription Order Form

Copy or detach and send to:

Jossey-Bass, A Wiley Imprint, 989 Market Street, San Francisco, CA 94103-1741

Call or fax toll-free: Phone 888-378-2537 6:30AM – 3PM PST; Fax 888-481-2665

Back issues: Please send me the following issues at $29 each.
(Important: please include series initials and issue number, such as YD100.)

_____

_____

_____

$ _____   Total for single issues

$ _____   Shipping charges:

	Surface	Domestic	Canadian
First item		$5.00	$6.00
Each add'l item		$3.00	$1.50

For next-day and second-day delivery rates, call the number listed above.

Subscriptions: Please __start __renew my subscription to *New Directions for Youth Development* for the year 2_____ at the following rate:

U.S.	__Individual $80	__Institutional $195
Canada	__Individual $80	__Institutional $235
All others	__Individual $104	__Institutional $269

**For more information about online subscriptions visit
www.interscience.wiley.com**

$ _____   Total single issues and subscriptions (Add appropriate sales tax for your state for single issue orders. No sales tax for U.S. subscriptions. Canadian residents, add GST for subscriptions and single issues.)

__Payment enclosed (U.S. check or money order only)
__VISA __MC __AmEx #_____ Exp. date _____

Signature _____ Day phone _____
__ Bill me (U.S. institutional orders only. Purchase order required.)

Purchase order # _____
                 Federal Tax ID13559302   **GST 89102 8052**

Name _____

Address _____

_____

Phone _____ E-mail _____

For more information about Jossey-Bass, visit our Web site at **www.josseybass.com**